WORKOUT & WORSHIP

8 STEPS TO PHYSICAL & SPIRITUAL HEALTH

EXERCISE
DEVOTION
PRAYER

Lazet Michaels Boatmon

www.LAZETLIFE.com

Workout & Worship
8 Steps to Physical & Spiritual Health

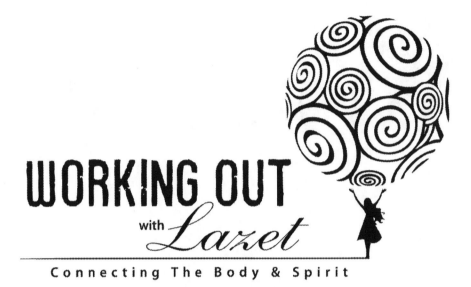

iUniverse books may be ordered through booksellers or by contacting:

iUniverse
1663 Liberty Drive
Bloomington, IN 47403
www.iuniverse.com
1-800-Authors (1-800-288-4677)

ISBN: 978-1-4401-6617-4 (pbk)
ISBN: 978-1-4401-6618-1 (ebook)

Printed in the United States of America

iUniverse rev. date: 12/01/10

Dedication

I would like to dedicate this book to my parents, Reverend James Shaffer and Reverend Maggie Shaffer. My dad is one hundred years old and my mom is eighty-four. Because they are in good health, we can enjoy each other, and I thank the Lord for that.

They exemplify pure health—mentally, physically, and spiritually. They love God, love God's people, and love life.

When I train them, they work out thirty minutes on bike and then I train them thirty minutes to tone, strengthen, and stretch.

They eat healthfully, juice, dress, and travel, and they love to cook a great feast and entertain. They want to see people enjoying life. What a great example of living life more abundantly

My mom is a self-taught herbologist. She taught herself the healing properties of different herbal teas. When I was growing up, people would give sick children to my mom, and she would keep them for about two to three weeks and hand them back to their parents, well.

My dad, a retired plumber, consistently eats small meals and loves to work. Just a couple of months ago my bathroom sink was stopped up. I was trying to wash my hair to prepare for a taping the next day. At ninety-nine years of age, he came downstairs and got under the sink, pulled all the pipes apart (took about ninety minutes), cleaned everything out, put all the pipes back together, and my totally stopped-up sink was flowing like a river.

My mom and dad are my examples, my motivation, and my encouragement. I praise the Lord that in my lifetime, I got a chance to see true worshippers of the living God living life to the fullest. My Dad's one hundredth birthday was February 13, 2010, and even if I had a thousand tongues, I could not express my thankfulness.

I thank you, Lord! Bless your Holy Name! Mom and Dad, I love you!

This book is also dedicated to my wonderful sister Diane Boatmon Fuller, who died on Pan Am 103. You were always my hero, but now you are a hero to the nation. I love you, girl!

And to my wonderful brothers Cannon and Calvin, who are not with us today. Calvin, you encouraged me to run. Remember, when I was ten years old, you used to run backward while I was hustling forward to keep up? You were truly my first running coach. Cannon, I remember when a group of us challenged each other after a party; we had been up all night, and we went to Belle Isle park and ran. Of the ten people, you were the third one to make it to the finish line … Amazing!

And to my wonderful, fun, and loving sisters and brothers whom I have the opportunity to hang out with every day—Marie, Louise, Michael, Joyce, and Chris—I decree and declare that we are all healed in every area of our lives in Jesus's name.

To my true partners and friends and *Working Out with Lazet*/Life Center staff, Reginald K. Pelzer, Vernon Isby, DiAnn Mason and Anita Stephens, I thank the Lord for you!

To my friends and family who have enjoyed and supported my television ministry, the *Working Out with Lazet* program, and my heart, which is those at the Life Center private fitness facility in Detroit. We have been through a lot together, but we are achieving incredible goals in weight loss and physical and spiritual health.

This book was written for "The Healing of the Nations"! Be an example and encourage somebody today!

Table of Contents

Foreword

God killed Goliath through David. God built an ark through Noah. God uses people to get what he wants. Without your health, Satan may rob you of the gift that God has given you. It is important to be strong and healthy enough to do what God has called us to do. When Satan comes against our bodies, he is attacking the temple of the Holy Spirit.

The National Institute of Health, the Centers for Disease Control and Prevention, and the American Heart Association say that our individual weight problems have become a national crisis. One hundred ninety million Americans are obese or overweight, which is two out of every three people.

John 10:10 kjv says, *"The thief cometh not but to steal, kill and destroy."* My testimony is that I lost my biological dad to a heart attack at the age of seventy. My favorite brother died of a heart attack in his early forties. Another brother died of a stroke in his early fifties. One of my best friends died of a blood clot in her legs just three years ago. She was in her early forties. Last year, I spoke to another friend of mine on Sunday, and he died on Monday of a heart attack at forty-two years of age. In my family we have a background of obesity, diabetes, cancer, high blood pressure, and cardiovascular disease. I made a decision when I was twelve years old to live a healthy lifestyle. Whatever age you are, it's not too late. As soon as you start walking or running while eating the proper diet, your blood pressure will lower. Ask any doctor. That is simply how God made our bodies … always to heal. Plus, my God can do anything but fail.

In Genesis 6:3 the Lord promises us 120 years. *"And the Lord said, My spirit shall not always strive with man, for that he also is flesh: yet his days shall be an hundred and twenty years."*

I want you to live a long life in good health. Please don't die this year! I hope this book and the "Working Out with Lazet" ministry will encourage you and your family and friends.

This book begins by explaining all the reasons why you should work out, which is the eight steps; then the posture for each basic exercise; four or five exercises for each major muscle group; then a fifteen-minute fast and fun workout; a full workout; and then a scripture and a prayer for each month to keep you encouraged in your workout for the full year.

My recommendation is to read the full book up to the first prayer, first. Go over the exercises to see which program would be best for you.

a. The fifteen-minute fast and fun

b. The full workout

c. Make up your own program from the exercises displayed (if you already work out).

Beginners, be careful with the different exercises, see the illustrated pictures, and read how to perform the exercises. Follow the form and the illustrations exactly. If you have issues with your knees, you do not want to perform the squats or lunges, but you can do the straight-leg exercises, abdominals, and upper-body exercises. Plus, you can always walk for your aerobic exercise, with your doctor's consent.

After you choose the exercise program that you would like, perform it every other day for three weeks and then build up over six to eight weeks to five times a week without weights. If you use weights, know that you are not supposed to perform the same exercise with weights two days in a row. You can perform upper-body one day and lower-body the next, or the front of your body one day and the back of your body the next. You can also split the body into parts—for example, legs and shoulders and arms one day, and chest and back the next.

As you are working out, remember to meditate on one scripture and one prayer for one month or four weeks. Most scripture references are from the King James version of the bible. Let this scripture and prayer led by the Holy Spirit get into your spirit and empower you to heal and change in Jesus name.

I love you and God bless you. I am looking forward to testimony. *"Be Strong in the Lord and in the power of his might"* (Ephesians 6:10). Jesus said, *"I am come that they might have life, and that more abundantly"* (John 10:10).

CHAPTER ONE

The Eight Steps

Chapter One: The Eight Steps

The Eight Steps

You can agree that the Lord wants to be in the middle of your marriage, your children, your relationships and friendships, in your work, in the midst of your dreams and goals. Well, folks, he wants to be a part of your workout, too! Many of you know this scripture: *"What? Know ye not that your body is the temple of the holy spirit? Therefore glorify God in your body and in your spirit"* (I Corinthians 6:19). Working out is a fine opportunity to glorify God in your body and your spirit simultaneously.

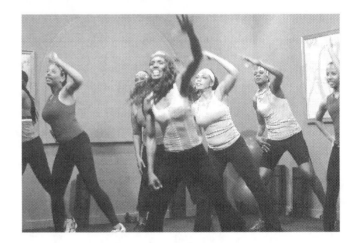

When I work out, I pray, worship, listen to the Word, and study scripture. I want to show you how to glorify God as you work out. I will express to you the importance of planting the seeds of nutrition and fitness in your life and how to begin. The seedtime word to remember is "discipline." I'm speaking directly to those who say, "I can't find the time to work out; my schedule is too busy"; "I start a program and then I get bored and stop"; I can't afford to or don't belong to a gym." Excuses, excuses! We have heard them all, and now is the time to plant the seeds of information to harvest a healthy body and a life of fitness. Okay, you busy people, how about a thirty- to forty-minute workout three to five times a week. And for those who don't belong to a gym: you don't need a gym. I am presenting to you a workout program that you can perform in the gym or at home … anywhere. With this program and healthy eating, in six to eight weeks you will look and feel great! But that is only the beginning. Remember, a healthy lifestyle (fitness and nutrition) is for a lifetime. And this book encourages a one-year plan of consistent programming in health, nutrition, and wellness through the Lord Jesus Christ. Now I would like to present eight steps to physical and spiritual health.

Step One: Make a Decision

We have forgotten about our health and nutrition and have filled those spaces in our lives with being busy. Most people today say that they don't have time to work out. We've filled our schedules with so many things that we truly do not have time unless we make the time. We are more concerned about money than health. We adorn the outside of our and our children's bodies with expensive sneakers, shoes, jewelry, clothing, houses, and cars. Gym classes have been taken out of the schools, and we have become what I call the "remote control generation" (will not get off the couch for anything). Whatever happened to eating dinner at the dinner table with the family at home? We are eating at fast-food places in the car at the drive-in window. The car has become the dinner table. We have all read that fast food is high-calorie, high-fat food with zero nutritional value—not good for us, and could be the reason for our illness—but we don't care.

We are so comfortable in our disease and obesity that we truly have to ask the question "Why work out?" even though we are twenty to one hundred pounds overweight. So we wait until we are sick and on our way to the emergency room to make a healthy lifestyle change and a **decision** … if we live to make that change. Today it seems that the threat of death is our only encouragement. A report from CBS news, "Battling Obesity in America," says that two out of every three Americans are overweight or obese. One hundred ninety million people in America are obese. The National Institute of Health says that obesity means having too much body fat. It is different from being overweight, which means weighing too much. Both terms mean that a person's weight is greater than what is considered healthy for his or her height. There are thirty diseases and conditions associated with obesity:

1. Coronary heart disease
2. Type 2 diabetes
3. Hypertension
4. Dyslipidemia
5. Stroke

6. Sleep Apnea
7. Pulmonary dysfunction
8. Gall bladder disease
9. Liver disease
10. Osteoarthritis
11. Gout
12. Some cancers—colon, endometrial, postmenopausal breast cancer
13. Menstrual irregularities
14. Polycystic ovary syndrome
15. Infertility
16. Gestational diabetes
17. Neural tube defects in offspring
18. Low-back pain
19. Increased risk of complications from anesthesia
20. Carpal tunnel syndrome
21. Venous insufficiency
22. Deep vein thrombosis
23. Poor wound healing
24. Psychosocial problems
25. Osteoporosis; obesity is protective
26. Stress incontinence and leaking urine
27. Prolapse
28. Esophageal reflux
29. Constipation
30. Tiredness

Chapter One: The Eight Steps

Well, working out was not designed for sick people. Working out was designed to strengthen our bodies for sports, athletics, and everyday life. Now, fortunately, we find that working out also helps to prevent disease and can help battle and manage diseases that we may already have. Remember: working out is for everyone. The Lord designed our bodies, shoulders, and hips to go in different directions; we were designed to run and jump, dance and walk long distances. Palms 150: 1–6 says, *"Praise ye the Lord. Praise God in his sanctuary: Praise him in the firmaments of his power. Praise him for his mighty acts: praise him according to his excellent greatness. Praise him with the sound of the trumpet: praise him with the psaltery and harp. Praise him with the timbrel and dance."* No wonder David danced his clothes off. To praise the Lord like this takes a lot of energy, vitality, health, wellness, and fitness. So again, I Corinthians 6:19 says, *"What? Know ye not that your body is the temple of the Holy Ghost which is in you, which ye have of God, and ye are not your own?"* Working out should be for the rest of your life. Make the decision.

- **See the doctor**
- **Take time**
- **Don't wait**
- **Choose a type of exercise**
- **Be encouraged**

See the doctor

Before you start any exercise program, it is important to see the doctor. In most cases, the doctor has already asked us to start an exercise program. Be sure you tell the doctor that you are planning to work out. The doctor may be able to encourage what type of exercise program you should begin. If you already work out, then it's good to know that you are healthy and that you can continue your program and maybe even intensify it. If you have issues with your shoulders, hips, knees, back, or any other physical restraints, then tell the doctor and get the issue resolved before starting any

Chapter One: The Eight Steps

exercise program. The doctor may recommend seeing a physical therapist first before beginning any exercise program. Listen to your doctor.

Again, I hear you say in your mind, *I don't have time.*

What you value, you make room for. The Bible says, *"I give you life and death, blessings and cursings, choose Life!"* Are you overweight? Do you have a disease? Do you want to end generational curses of sickness, disease, depression, etc? Do you want to prevent disease? Do you want to be fit and happy and press forward to ultimate health and strength? Do you want to achieve your purpose? Then it's time to work out. Put in the forefront of your mind the reason that you are making the decision to work out. You have a reason. Let this be your motivation. Write it down and make it plain. Habakak 2:2 says, *"Write the vision, and make it plain upon tables, that he may run that readeth it."*

Don't wait

Work on the offensive, not the defensive, working ahead of circumstances and situations that may come upon you. This is my reason for working out. I pray for health, healing, and a long life, now, in Jesus's name. I eat fruits and vegetables, take herbs, and consume all that God has left for the healing of the nations. I'm not a vegetarian, but I was once, for two years. I'm not saying that everyone should be vegetarian, but in order to increase your health, it is important to eat fruit and vegetables every day. Genesis 1:29 says, *"And God said behold, I have given you every herb bearing seed, which is upon the face of all the earth, and every tree, in the which is the fruit of a tree yielding seed, to you it shall be for meat."* Start eating right by adding at least a salad and two pieces of fruit every day and start at least to walk at a track, the mall, at home on a treadmill or at the gym, or perhaps even undertake a full workout program from this book today. Every day is crucial. The Bible says that every day you have the opportunity to choose life or death, blessings or cursings. Choose life!

Choose a type of exercise

Choose an exercise that you enjoyed when you were a child. Did you like walking, running, jumping rope, cycling, swimming, boxing, skating, dancing? If you choose to work with a fitness professional or trainer, then, depending on the trainer you choose, you can work out with resistance balls, medicine balls, dumbbells and functional training. You can also do yoga, pilates, biking, dancing, cardio classes, and more. Are you going to train at home or are you going to purchase a gym membership? Are you going to train alone or with a partner, group of friends, class, or trainer?

Exercise is not supposed to be stressful and hard. Yes, working out is supposed to challenge you, eventually, but in the beginning remember to keep it light and choose only those things that you enjoy. You will then continue your workouts and be consistent. Consistency is the key. If you work out three to five times a week, you will achieve very noticeable results. When you receive results, you are encouraged, and when you are encouraged, you keep on going.

Be encouraged

Working out is fun. It's so much fun to be able to walk and run and jump and chase after children, to be able to bend and stretch, to be strong enough to help someone physically, to be able to pick up your children, to be able to walk up a flight of stairs without being winded, to dance at a party all night long, or how about running around the church for the victory as many times as the Holy Spirit will allow? Many believe that working out is a thing of the past or the thought of working out is someone jumping up and down, winded and not having a good time. That is not proper exercise. Working out is fun and controlled, and it feels real good! If you do not feel good even if you are challenged during or after working out, then you are not working out properly, and you need to get information and instruction on how you should proceed.

So many say, "I feel and look fine. Why should I work out?"

Be honest with yourself: if you are not working out, you feel sluggish, tired, you have that little twinge in your hip or that little thing in your knee, or maybe it's your back. And of course your family and friends and relationships are totally stressing you out. If you are eating, drinking, or smoking too much, you are adding to the dilemma.

Chapter One: The Eight Steps

Also know that the environment is no longer conducive to good health. The pollution in the air, the chemicals in the food that we eat, and the normal stresses of life will degenerate your health. In order to keep anything in good shape, including your car or your house, you must do the maintenance work. Do those things that will increase your health. Your body will work like a dream, look goo,d and, with the word of the Lord, you will surely be on your way to living a long, healthy, and prosperous life. So, again, "I feel and look fine. Why should I work out?"

1. For preventative reasons. To fight disease.
2. To fight muscle, joint, and bone weaknesses.
3. To fight stress and depression.
4. To keep the blood flowing and your circulatory system healthy, which will raise your metabolism.
5. To look beautiful or handsome in clothing, glorifying God to others around you, being in good health, which is ministry.
6. To pray, worship, and praise like never before.

So yes! Be encouraged! You can do it!

I Corinthians 3:16–17 says, *"Know ye not that ye are the temple of God, and that the Spirit of God dwelleth in you? If any may defile the temple of God, him shall God destroy; for the temple of God is holy, which temple ye are."*

Step Two: Set Goals

Exercise, health, and wellness is the talk of the country; it's unfortunate that talking won't help you to lose weight … it's all about executing … making that move. Like the Nike commercial says, "Just do it!" After you have truly made the decision to work out and eat healthfully, then it is time to set your goals. Is your goal to lose weight? How much? Conquer a disease? Play with your children? Are you striving for ultimate health and physical appearance? Are you looking to run a marathon? To bicycle a marathon? When will you work out? What days and where? Until these questions are explored and answered, your decision to work out may not be executed. Notice that every day there will be a voice telling you that you do not need to work out, you've gone this long without it, and the voice says that you are hopeless or maybe the voice says, "There isn't anything wrong with you, why go? Aren't you tired?" The voice says that there's always tomorrow. Sit down today and start tomorrow … have that pork and cake today, and start tomorrow. I pull down that stronghold of laziness and indecisiveness in Jesus's name!

- **What is your goal?**
- **Planning your workout**

Is your goal to lose weight?

How much weight does the doctor say you should lose? Don't be alarmed. Set small goals. Do you want to lose ten pounds, fifty pounds, one hundred pounds? All right, then. Write it down and make it plain (Habakak 2:2).

Stay focused on your goal, and commit to the first three weeks of your one-year plan. Begin by performing a cardiovascular workout (which is working out your heart and lungs and burning fat calories). Biking, walking, running, jumping rope, skating, aerobics classes, or kickboxing are examples of cardiovascular workouts and should be performed twenty to thirty minutes every other day starting out, eventually building up to sixty minutes five times a week.

Chapter One: The Eight Steps

If you can only walk five or ten minutes at a time, start off slow and work out for five minutes—or whatever small amount—every other day. As the days progress, you will progress. Cardiovascular workouts will become easier. It takes three weeks to acclimate to a fitness program, so even though you may feel uncomfortable in the beginning, after three weeks, you will feel great.

Keep a journal of what you are eating, and be honest. Statistics show a 90 percent success rate of taking it off and keeping it off when a journal is used. Take your weight and your measurements every two weeks to track your progress. Measure your body fat percent every six weeks. Also record in the journal your thoughts, emotions, and victories. Never take your victories for granted. Many times we overlook our victories and quickly forget our progress and become discouraged. You can safely and effectively lose two to three pounds a week, which is approximately twelve pounds a month by eating nutritiously and working out three to five times a week.

Check your BMI, which is your Body Mass Index. It is your weight relative to your height. BMI is a quick and easy method for determining what your weight should be. To assess weight relative to height (BMI), divide body weight (in kilograms) by height (in meters squared). (See the BMI chart on page 125.) Normal weight range is 19–24.9, overweight is 25–30, and obesity is above 30. The most recent studies are putting more emphasis on the waistline. The New York Times reports that Dr. Corner, obesity specialist at Columbia University, says that an overweight woman with a waistline of thirty-five inches or larger, or an overweight man with at least a forty-inch waist is at increased risk for diabetes and heart disease.

Is your goal to conquer a disease?

Do you have high blood pressure? Diabetes? Cardiovascular disease? Cancer? If so, keep in mind that it usually takes thirty minutes of cardio workouts at least five times a week to impact disease conditions. After you get clearance from your doctor to work out, make sure that you consult with a fitness professional who can design a program for you, and keep in touch with your physician to monitor your progress. Following are some tips on working out for special populations.

Chapter One: The Eight Steps

Cardiovascular disorders

Low-intensity endurance exercise, such as low-impact aerobics, walking, swimming, or stationary cycling should be the primary exercise mode.

Avoid isometric exercises because they can dramatically raise blood pressure and the work of the heart. Perform low-resistance workouts with a high number of repetitions. Total duration should gradually be increased to twenty or thirty minutes of continuous or interval training, plus additional time for warm-up and cool down activities. Frequency should be three to five times per week.

Hypertension

The American Council on Exercise (ACE) says that hypertension is one of the most prevalent chronic diseases in the United States. The ACE also says that as many as fifty million Americans have chronically elevated blood pressure greater than 140/90 mmHg, or are taking antihypertensive medication. Exercise is recognized as an important part of therapy for controlling hypertension. Regular aerobic exercise reduces both systolic and diastolic blood pressure. Since many hypertensive individuals are obese and have coronary artery disease (CAD) risk factors, non-drug therapy is usually the first line of treatment. This therapy will usually include weight reduction, salt restriction, and increased physical activity. Endurance exercise such as low-impact aerobics, walking, and swimming should be the primary exercise mode. Hypertensives should exercise at least four times per week.

Diabetes

Before beginning an exercise program, diabetics should speak with their physician or diabetes educator to develop a program of diet, exercise, and medication. Diabetics should perform endurance activities such as walking, swimming, and cycling. Frequency should be four to five days a week for IDDM (insulin-dependent diabetes mellitus) and five to seven days a week for NIDDM (non-insulin-dependent diabetes mellitus). Some clients may need to start out with several shorter daily sessions. Individuals with IDDM should gradually work up to twenty to thirty minutes per session. For individuals with NIDDM, forty to sixty minutes is recommended.

Chapter One: The Eight Steps

Asthma

Asthmatics should have a bronchiodilating inhaler with them at all times and be instructed to use it at the first sign of wheezing. Dynamic exercise, walking, cycling, and swimming are good choices for one with an asthmatic condition. It is important to work out at least three to four times per week. Individuals with low functional capacities or those who experience shortness of breath during prolonged exercise may benefit from intermittent exercise (two ten-minute sessions). It is important to do a longer, gradual warm-up and cool down (longer than ten minutes). Gradually increase total exercise duration to twenty to forty-five minutes.

Osteoporosis

Resistance training is an important component in the prevention of osteoporosis. The greater the physical stress and compression on a bone, the greater the rate of bone deposition (this is why weight-bearing exercise is recommended). Do not perform high impact aerobics.

Arthritis

Non-weight-bearing activities such as cycling, warm-water aquatic programs, and swimming are preferred because they reduce joint stress. Recommended water temperature is 83 degrees F (28° C) to 88 degrees F (31° C).

Arthritic individuals should be encouraged to exercise at least four to five times per week. Perform long, gradual warm-up and cool-down periods (longer than ten minutes). Initial exercise sessions should last no longer than ten to fifteen minutes.

Cancer

The following is information from the American College of Sports Medicine Roundtable on Exercise Guidelines for Cancer Survivors:

> In 2009, the American Cancer Society (ACS) estimated that there were nearly 1.5 million new cases of cancer diagnosed in the United States and just more than 500,000 people who died from the disease. Currently, there are close to 12 million cancer survivors in the United States and this number grows each year.

Chapter One: The Eight Steps

In the last two decades it has become clear that exercise plays a vital role in cancer prevention and control. There is growing evidence suggesting that exercise decreases the risk of many of cancers and data to support the premise that exercise may extend life for breast and colon cancer survivors are emerging. The focus here is on the influence of regular exercise on the health, quality of life (QOL), and psychosocial well-being of cancer survivors after diagnosis. Studies reviewed have hypothesized that some of the psychological and physiological challenges faced by cancer survivors can be prevented, attenuated or treated through exercise.

These are the existing recommendations for exercise from the ACSM and the American Heart Association, the ACS, and the U.S. Department of Health and Human Services. The recent U.S. DHHS guidelines indicate that, when individuals with chronic conditions such as cancer are unable to meet the stated recommendation on the basis of their health status, "[T]hey should be as physically active as their abilities and conditions allow." An explicit recommendation was made to "avoid inactivity," and it was clearly stated that "Some physical activity is better than none." The U.S. DHHS guideline for aerobic activity focused on overall weekly activity of 150 minutes of moderate-intensity exercise or 75 minutes of vigorous-intensity exercise or an equivalent combination.

Guidance for strength training is to perform two to three weekly sessions that include exercises for major muscle groups. Flexibility guidelines are to stretch major muscle groups and tendons on days that other exercises are performed.

Planning your workout

It is important to plan what time, what days, and where you are going to work out. I bring up this subject matter because many of us say that we are going to start to working out—even today—but do not have a plan. Many times in our minds we've fooled ourselves into thinking that we tried, but it wasn't successful when, realistically, we didn't plan; therefore, there was no action.

In choosing what time to work out, choose whether you are going to work out in the morning or the evening. I like to encourage the morning because we do not have

Chapter One: The Eight Steps

to deal with all the issues of the day, such as what to eat, what time, and how much. When working out early, it is important first to drink water and orange juice and then eat something very light like an apple, a small bowl of cereal or oatmeal, a granola bar, or yogurt and banana. Usually early in the morning we haven't had a chance to get hungry, so a light breakfast is satisfying. For many our highest energy is in the morning, which can make a workout most enjoyable. If the evening is better for you, make sure that you eat two to three hours before the workout if you eat heavily. Eating something light before a workout usually gets the best results because it gives you pure energy without the extra. Eating heavily before a workout can make you feel heavy, bloated, and tired and not able to perform well. If you eat two to three hours before a workout, there is time for the food to be digested.

In choosing what days to work out, if you are a beginner, choose every other day s uch as Monday, Wednesday, and Friday or Tuesday, Thursday, and Saturday. It is important to have the days and times already established as part of your goal and to stick to them.

In choosing where to work out, just make the decision whether it will be the park, the gym, or home. If you find a partner to work out with, then there is someone to keep you accountable, and you can encourage each other.

Nutrition and exercise go together

If you are consuming large numbers of calories and working out, you will feel better and get stronger and healthier, but you will not lose weight. If you are eating nutritiously but not working out, you may lose some weight but without physical exercise, it is easy to gain it back. To be physically fit is not just about losing weight. It's important for your muscles to get stronger so that you can run and walk and stand and sit and push and pull. It's important to strengthen your heart and lungs so that you can run and walk (run and not be weary; walk and not faint) and also to prevent heart attacks and strokes. It's important to do weight-bearing exercise to tone muscles and strengthen your bones to prevent osteoporosis and to stretch for flexibility. Flexibility helps to prevent injury to the joints and muscles, and it also helps in standing and sitting and moving and bending and reaching. So it is important to not only lose weight but to be healthy and fit.

Nutrition Tips

Do not diet. Dieting does not work. You lose weight and gain it all back and more. Instead, change your way of eating. IDEA Health and Fitness Association says "Avoid dieting. Don't try to deprive yourself of any one food group … choose a well balanced natural foods diet, which will provide the structural components for protein synthesis

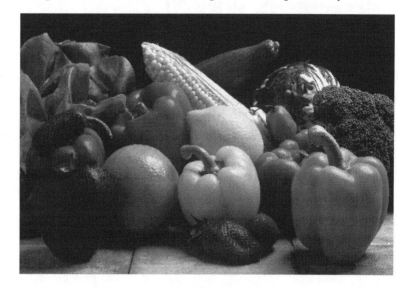

and supply adequate energy. Rather than dieting, restrict your food portions by using measuring cups and smaller plates and quit eating once you are naturally satiated." Practice eating nutritiously.

Do not drink soda or diet soda; drink peppermint tea or green tea, which raises your metabolism and keeps your circulatory system going. Drink at least eight glasses of water a day. Water keeps you energized, and it aids in keeping your metabolism high. When working out, it is important to drink at least four ounces of water every fifteen minutes.

Following are some examples of nutritious meals.

Breakfast Sample
- Oatmeal and blueberries or strawberries, one to two slices turkey bacon— sweeten with agave, honey, or stevia; peppermint tea, green tea
- One or two boiled eggs, one half cup of grits, one to two slices turkey bacon
- Cereal, one half cup of almond milk or soy milk, half a banana
- Yogurt, fruit/granola

Chapter One: The Eight Steps

Lunch Sample
- Open-face tuna, turkey, or chicken breast sandwich (one slice of bread), fruit, yogurt, or granola bar for snack
- Tuna (solid white in water), dry, one half cup rice, salad
- Chicken, salmon, tuna, or shrimp salad

Dinner Sample
- Tuna, chicken, salmon, or shrimp salad, etc.
- Tilapia or salmon, small red potato, salad
- Chicken breast, spinach or greens, small yam
- One medium-large yam and salad

Six Classes of Nutrients and Major Functions

1. **Protein:** Builds and repairs body tissue; major component of enzymes, hormones, and antibodies.

2. **Carbohydrate:** Provide a major source of fuel to the body; provide dietary fibers.

3. **Lipids:** Chief form of stored energy in the body; insulate and protect vital organs, and provide fat-soluble vitamins.

4. **Vitamins:** Help promote and regulate various chemical reactions and bodily processes; do not yield energy themselves but participate in releasing energy from food.

5. **Minerals:** Enable enzymes to function; are a component of hormones and a part of bone and nerve impulses.

6. **Water:** Enables chemical reactions to occur; about 70 percent of the body is composed of water; essential for life, as we cannot store it or conserve it.

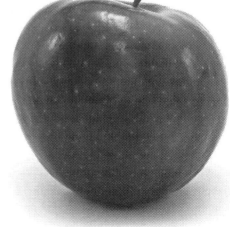

The Importance of Water

Water regulates body temperature, transports nutrients and oxygen to cells, removes waste, cushions joints, and protects organs and tissues. Dr. Don Colbert's book *"Eat This and Live!"* documents that you can live five to seven weeks without food, but the average adult can last no longer than five days without water.

According to Dr. Colbert:

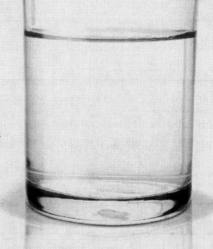

- Your body is about 70 percent water
- Your muscles are 75 percent water
- Your brain is 85 percent water
- Your blood is 82 percent water
- Your bones are 25 percent water

When asked how much water you should drink, Dr. Colbert says to take your weight in pounds and divide by two. The result is how many ounces of water you should drink daily. The best times to drink water are: you should start with eight to sixteen ounces a half hour before breakfast, and a couple of hours after breakfast it is good to drink eight to sixteen ounces of water..

2 hours after dinner, have another 8 ounces and another before bedtime unless you have a hiatal hernia, reflux disease, enlarged prostate, or frequent urination during the night. In those cases do not drink anything else after dinner.

Thirty minutes before your evening meal, drink sixteen to twenty-four ounces. (If lunch is your big meal, drink sixteen to twenty-four ounces before that meal.) Afterward you will not usually eat as much.

Two hours after dinner, have another eight ounces and another before bedtime, unless you have a hiatal hernia, reflux disease, an enlarged prostate, or frequent urination during the night. In those cases, do not drink anything else after dinner.

Chapter One: The Eight Steps

Overindulgence in fat, sugar, and sodium are risk factors in the leading causes of death in the United States. The federal government issued the Dietary Guidelines—seven principles that all Americans should know in order to make wise food choices.

- Eat a variety of foods.
- Balance the food you eat with physical activity to maintain or improve your weight.
- Choose a diet low in total fat, saturated fat, and cholesterol.
- Choose a diet with plenty of vegetables, fruits, and grain products.
- Choose a diet moderate in sugar.
- Choose a diet moderate in salt and sodium.
- Avoid alcoholic beverages.

Simply concentrate on eating frequent healthy meals and small portions. Eat at least one salad every day and add at least two pieces of fruit every day to your diet. I encourage you to eat organic. Organic means that the fruits and vegetables have not been sprayed with pesticides and chemicals to increase growth. They are naturally grown. Fruits and vegetables encourage your body to eliminate, which is the key to health and losing weight. Too many carbohydrates and white sugars will bloat you and slow down the elimination process.

Add green juice from an organic health food store to your diet two or three times a week. This can include collards, kale, spinach, cucumbers, parsley, bok choy, etc. This food is from the Lord. Eat four to five meals a day. Eat real food, not fast food, which carries approximately 2,000–5,000 or more calories per sitting and has no nutritional value whatsoever.

Chapter One: The Eight Steps

There is a sweetener craze going on in this country. The best sweeteners to use are natural sweeteners such as brown sugar, honey, organic maple syrup, agave, and stevia. Artificial sweeteners are either unsafe or poorly tested. (For more information on artificial sweeteners, see the Web site www.anhcampaign.org.) Do not drink diet sodas and try to avoid regular sodas and sweet teas. I call these beverages "diabetes juices."

In Dr. Colbert's book *"Eat This and Live,"* he states that many people think diet sodas help them lose weight, but one study showed otherwise. A study covering eight years of collected data showed that your risk of becoming overweight by drinking one to two cans of soda per day is 32.8%, but your risk increases to 54.5% if you drink one or two cans of diet soda instead.

I encourage foods and beverages that are natural. I do not encourage fast foods or artificial colors and flavorings.

Ask the Lord to give you the strength and the desire to eat right. Let's face facts: we all cheat every once in a while, and it's okay. But it's important to be disciplined to eat healthfully on a daily basis. It's the daily habits that can make you or break you. Find foods that are healthy that you really enjoy. Again, I can not stress the importance of keeping a journal of everything that you are eating. Statistics show that there is a 90 percent success rate in losing weight and keeping it off if you keep a journal of what you are eating. Look at your journal and discuss it with a nutritionist or dietitian or your trainer and make healthy adjustments.

Now that the seed has been sown for the desire to work out and the desire to eat right, we are on the right track.

Step Three: Get a Trainer

I encourage all who can afford it to hire a trainer. Most of us can't afford not to. It is important to have a safe workout program that works every muscle group in your body. Strengthening some muscles and not others can cause an imbalance in your body, which can cause injury. A good trainer will design a well-balanced program for you where you are working every muscle group. If you can't afford a trainer, then make sure you get a trainer's advice.

- **Is your trainer certified?**
- **Get an initial consultation**

Check to see whether the trainer is certified. It is important to get a trainer who is skillful in designing a program that addresses your particular needs. A certified trainer follows the guidelines of a doctor and physical therapist. A certified trainer is taught never to diagnose a condition. Unless your trainer is also an MD, don't look to your trainer to be your doctor.

If you are a member of a gym, then get advice or an initial consultation with a trainer on staff. Most gyms offer this service at no cost to familiarize you with their equipment. Take advantage of this service.

A personal trainer should be chosen to partner with you, to assist you in achieving your healthy goals. Your goals must be realistic. For example, everyone wants to look like Beyonce in six weeks. For some that may be a realistic goal, and for most it is not—depending on how much you need to lose or gain, what you eat, how strong you are, how energetic you are, and how motivated you are. I encourage my clients to be the very best you that you can ever be. If you are motivated enough, within a certain amount of time everyone you know will be trying to look like you! If your trainer is more motivated than you, then you may not achieve any of your goals. You as a client must be motivated and consistent and partner with your trainer in following his or her instructions in order to achieve the healthy goals set for you.

Step Four: Press Forward

The No. 1 issue in keeping a consistent exercise program where you get results is showing up. When you get to the gym, you are always glad that you did. As I mentioned before, there are always many voices in your head trying to convince you not to go.

This is how you win! Do not let anything stop you from working out. I call it pressing forward. Tell all your friends and family where you will be for that one hour three to five times a week.

I recommend that the day before your workout you put out everything you need, which should include the outfit that you will wear, your sneakers, and your gym bag. I always like to keep a bottle of water and an apple and a granola bar in my bag. When we are rushing we often forget to eat and then find ourselves at the fast-food drive-in.

If you are working out at home, have your DVDs set aside or your music picked out the day before. Wake up early enough to catch the *"Working Out with Lazet"* exercise, health, and wellness program or any other exercise program and make sure that you begin the workout at the top of the program, which usually includes a warm-up and a stretch. Don't miss the first five minutes of the workout. The first five minutes prepare your body for the rest of the workout. Our bodies need to be warmed up before a stretch, and the stretches at the beginning and especially at the end of a workout are crucial. Don't forget to stretch! And press forward!

Philippians 3:13–14: *"Brethren, I count not myself to have apprehended: but this one thing I do, forgetting those things which are behind, and reaching forth unto those things which are before, I press toward the mark for the prize of the high calling of God in Christ Jesus."*

Tips on how or when to start

Do you have any issues with your back, knees, hips, shoulders, joints, etc.? If you have any of these issues, run, do not walk, to your doctor and/or physical therapist and get them resolved. If you do not get your issues resolved, then you may have to live a

Chapter One: The Eight Steps

sedentary lifestyle for the rest of your life … and that would not be good because you are still young and full of energy (smile). You may not want to start a jogging program unless your doctor or physical therapist releases you to do so. Your issue could get worse and possibly put you in a position where you will not be able to walk without pain.

In order to plant good seeds of exercise, health and wellness, you must address your physical issues and ask your doctor to give you a written release to work out. (If you have had injuries and you are now cleared to work out, consult with a personal trainer who can speak with your doctor or physical therapist and lead you to a strengthening program designed just for you.) Ask your doctor what exercises you should do and which ones you should avoid. After you get a release from your doctor or physical therapist, you are ready to plant good seeds in good ground. Now it's time to work out!

Okay, you busy professionals or moms and dads who only have a limited amount of time. Try a half hour of cardio plus five minutes of stretching every other day early in the morning. If you start early, then you won't have to worry about what and when to eat, and other emotional matters of the day. Eat a piece of fruit (an apple, for example, providing fiber and pectin), or maybe a small bowl of cereal or a yogurt. That's all you need early in the morning to get started. Five, six, or seven in the morning will allow you to get up early enough to work out for thirty to forty-five minutes and then go to work. (If you can only do evenings, that is okay.) Start with cardio. You can either fast-walk or run or jump rope or bike. Take the clothes off your stationary bike or step machine, dance around the room, jog in place, shadow or kickbox, exercise with the "Working Out with Lazet" DVD, etc. Again, cardio helps to build your heart and lung muscles and keep the blood flowing through your veins.

Step Five: Be Consistent

Yes, now you have pressed forward with your program and, as you know, it is easier to obtain than to maintain. Working out one or two days is easy. But in order to achieve great results you must be consistent. We consistently eat poorly, and we are very consistent at not doing anything—that is, living a sedentary lifestyle. Just know that it is important to work out for the rest of your life. Our first goal is the first three to four weeks, and our second goal is one year.

- **Discipline**
- **Program**

Weeks one to three

Consistency, along with "discipline," is the key. You don't have to work out for long hours to get results. If you are a beginner, start with cardio only and concentrate on eating healthfully for the first three weeks. Your initial goal should be twenty to thirty minutes, but if you can only perform for five to ten minutes, then stay right there for the full three weeks. It takes three weeks for your body to acclimate to a program. So your body may initially feel like it's saying "No," but your spirit says "Yes!"

I Corinthians 9:26 says, *"Therefore I do not run like a man running aimlessly; I do not fight like a man beating the air. No, I beat my body and make it my slave so that after I have preached to others, I myself will not be disqualified for the prize."*

Week four to five

Add on resistance training, which is your squats and abdominal work, etc., for fifteen minutes. You have the choice to work out with or without weights. If you are short on time, cut down the cardio to twenty minutes and add on the fifteen-minute resistance training. Then your workout will be a total of forty minutes, including your stretch. For those with a full hour, keep your thirty-minute cardio and add on calisthenics or resistance training for the extra fifteen minutes, and, including your stretch, you have a

Chapter One: The Eight Steps

fifty-minute workout. For those who love to work out and have always had a program, use the full hour or more: thirty to sixty minutes of cardio and twenty to thirty minutes of resistance training and a five-minute stretch. Always stretch!

This is a perfect program for you because while you are doing your cardio (for example, bike) you can put the stationary bike right in front of the TV and watch your favorite preaching DVD.

My pastor says, "Change is the process of maturation" and "The only constant in life is change." So it's time to do this!

Turn your radio on to a Christian station or turn on your iPod and get on your treadmill or your bike, or get your jump rope. You can Workout & Worship like me. I run outside early in the morning, and I say, "Lord, thank you for the healthy function of my heart and lungs, thank you, Lord, for strengthening my hips and knees and joints, for you are Jehovah Rapha, my healer, and Jehovah Shamma God with me. I can't make it to six miles without you, Lord, and no weapon formed against me shall prosper!"

You can definitely worship and pray and give praise and thanksgiving as you work out. The time will pass quickly and your day will be blessed. Your family will be whole and you can pray for the world. So try it! Workout & Worship!

Week six

Starting in week six, add five to ten minutes of cardio if your schedule allows. Stick to this program plan for another six weeks. Following, in chapter four, is the fifteen-minute workout, and in chapter five is the full workout. If you have any trouble following these diagrams, then get the companion "Working Out with Lazet" DVD. Follow the program, and imitate the form exactly, and you are on your way to a fit and healthy lifestyle.

Personal tip

I like to work out in the morning. I run at either six or seven in the morning, four to six miles, on average. I do forty to sixty minutes of cardio (running), four to five times

Chapter One: The Eight Steps

a week, and then I do a half-hour weight training or calisthenics program three times a week. On average, I work out three times a week for about an hour and a half and one to two times for forty minutes, and I take two days off. I enjoy morning exercise because I don't have to be too concerned about what I eat, and the morning energy is the best energy of the day.

Summary

Weeks one to three: cardio only

Weeks four to five: Day 1, cardio; Day 2, cardio and resistance; Day 3, cardio; Day 4, resistance; Day 5, cardio and resistance; Days 6 and 7, off.

Week six: Day 1, cardio and resistance, Day 2, cardio, Day 3, off; Day 4, cardio and resistance; Day 5, cardio; Day 6, cardio and resistance; Day 7, off.

Chapter One: The Eight Steps

Step Six: Keep a Journal

Keeping a journal is key. In his book The Fat Smash Diet, Dr. Ian Smith states that there is a 90 percent success rate in taking the weight off and keeping it off when you journal. It is also good to journal about what you are feeling and the progress you have made in your workout. When you are working out, there is always progress. The progress may be as simple as "I'm feeling great"; "I ran five extra minutes today"; "I did an extra push-up"; "I lost three pounds!"

- **Be honest about food**
- **Keep track of your workouts**

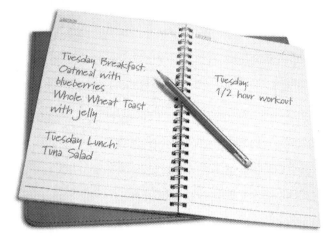

Being honest about what you are eating is key because that way you can detail your weight gains and losses, and determine which combination of foods works best for you. Just remember that the journal is for you; don't cheat yourself.

The journal also makes it easy for your nutritionist, doctor, or trainer to help you determine which combinations of food will help you to lose weight or lower your body fat percentage. My clients turn in a journal every week, and we talk food all the time.

If you do happen to have lapses in your program, remember not to beat yourself up. If you want chocolate cake or a bag of chips one day, go for it and write it down. Enjoy the chocolate cake. Maybe your body was craving sweet or salt, and we have those days. Just know that if you have these days too often, you may not achieve your weight-loss goals. Falling off your nutritional program for one day is not the problem. Problems begin when most times you are not eating nutritiously.

Step Seven: Keep a Good Attitude

Do not take the troubles of the day with you when you work out. Let your workout be your escape. Family issues, children, school, work, and any thoughts that cause you stress should not be taken with you when you work out. If you must think on certain issues, it is important to "work out and worship" alone with just you and God. Speak to the Lord, make your request known, worship him, and thank him for all he has done and all that he will do. Just worship him in your own words just for being God, your Savior. From this experience, this book, Work Out and Worship, was written. Believe me, the issues of the day will be resolved, and the Lord will give you a plan to answer your needs if you pray in Jesus's Name.

Here's what the Apostle Paul had to say regarding what we should think about. This is a mental exercise: *"Finally, brethren, whatsoever things are true, whatsoever things are honest, whatsoever things are just, whatsoever things are pure, whatsoever things are lovely, whatsoever things are of good report; if there be any virtue, and if there be any praise, think on these things"* (Philippians 4:8).

When you work out, just as when you party or hang out or vacation, leave your cares behind. Let working out be the best experience of your day. Listen to your favorite music. Listen to or watch something that will make you laugh or smile. Think of the ocean, a sunrise or sunset, a funny incident. Think of the goodness of God and what he has done for you. How he woke you up this morning. Think on how the Lord has kept you.

Think about the day that you will reach your goal. It will be like when Abraham received the promise. Notice that it says, *"And so after he had patiently endured, he obtained the promise"* (Hebrews 6:15).

Be patient with yourself. You will achieve your goals if you do not quit or faint. You spent a while eating bad food and avoiding exercise by living a sedentary lifestyle, and you patiently and consistently got yourself in the condition that you are in. Give yourself more than one day or one week to achieve your goals. Your goal is to work out consistently for one year. If you are consistent, each week you will see changes and/or

Chapter One: The Eight Steps

feel better, and you will consistently get stronger and healthier.

Hebrews 6:11 (amplified), *"But we do (strongly and earnestly) desire for each of you to show the same diligence and sincerity (all the way through) in realizing and enjoying the full assurance and development of (your) hope until the end."*

Take this message seriously by following through on your program. It is so easy to begin, but it takes great courage to finish. In the beginning, we are usually so excited, but when our emotions wear off, and it seems as though it may be hard work sometimes, we find out what it takes to truly succeed. Just remember that your body was designed to move and run and jump and dance and stretch. Be a person who does succeed and finishes well!

Chapter One: The Eight Steps

Step Eight: Workout

These are basic exercises that must be performed accurately. Then it will be easier to perform other creative movements working the upper and lower body together. You can perform each exercise with or without weights. Start with light weights such as two, three, or four pounds for women and five, eight, or ten pounds for men.

- Squat exercise

- Lunge exercise

- Tricep press exercise

- Rowing exercise

- Bicep curl exercise

- Abdominal exercise

- Push Up exercise

- Lateral side raise exercise

- Rear leg raise exercise

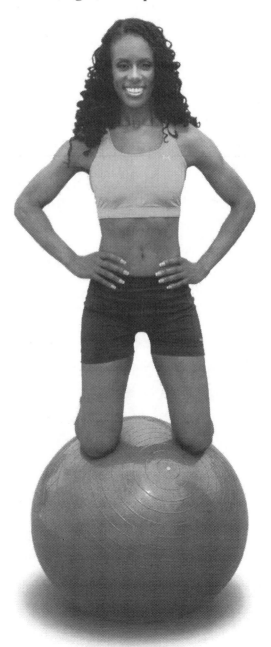

CHAPTER TWO

Basic Exercises

Chapter Two: Basic Exercises

Basic Exercises

Posture

When you are working out, posture and alignment are very important. With proper posture and alignment, you can target the muscle group you intend to develop and achieve incredible results. The targeted muscle and joint can be developed and toned properly, which will protect you from injury. Incorrect posture and alignment can cause injury.

Make sure that you stand as tall as you can, with feet parallel, holding your stomach in (continue to breathe), shoulders back, chest out, neck relaxed, chin level and forward. Imagine a string going through the center of your body pulling you up to the ceiling.

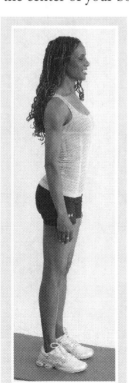

Arms are natural at your sides. Inhale deep breaths through your mouth and exhale. Inhale and exhale five times. Enjoy the feeling of proper alignment and practice utilizing it with all your exercises and in everyday life.

Chapter Two: Basic Exercises

Squat Assessment

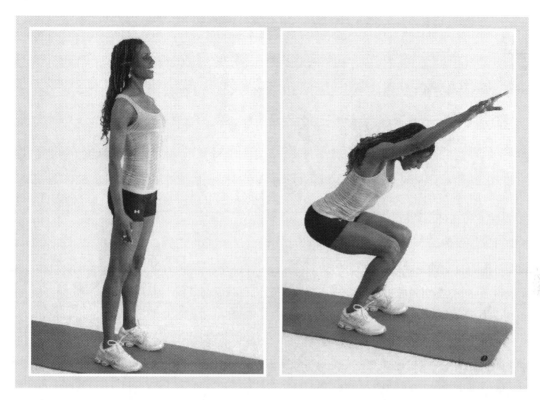

Squats are a basic movement. This squat assessment is your goal to reach for. There are many times a day when you will have to squat, such as sitting down, picking up packages, getting in and out of the car, playing with children, etc. Reaching is also a basic movement, as, for example, when you get items out of high cabinets, bookshelves, and the like.

If your arms will not reach the sides of your ears when you are performing a squat, then your arms and shoulders are too tight and need stretching.

To perform a correct squat:

1. Make sure your knees do not come together
2. Make sure your knees do not turn out
3. Make sure your knees do not go past your toes

Your trainer will usually give you a squat assessment to assess your strengths and weaknesses.

Basic Exercises

Squat

Quadriceps, Gluteals and Hamstrings – Start in a standing position with your feet hip-width apart, bend your knees, and sit back on your hips, pretending that you are sitting in a chair, and then return to a standing position. (If you have problems with squatting, then put a chair behind you, tap the edge of the chair with your buttocks, and return to a standing position.)

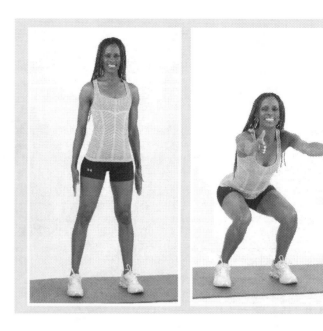

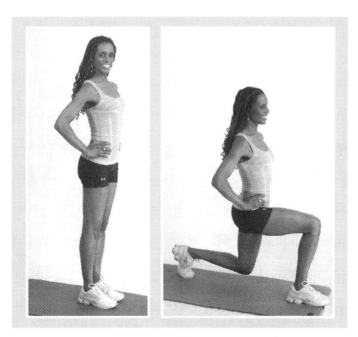

Lunge

Quadriceps, Gluteals, Hamstrings – Start in a standing position with your feet approximately two inches apart. Step forward with your right leg, bending so that the front leg is in a ninety-degree angle and then return your right leg to its original standing position. Change legs.

Chapter Two: Basic Exercises

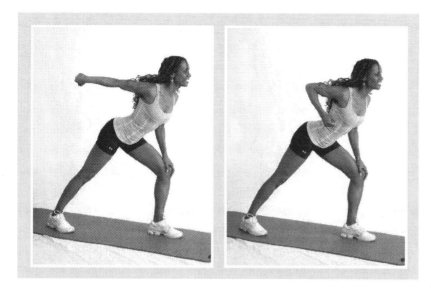

Triceps

Triceps – The front leg is bent and the back leg is straight. Weight is centered, so there is no pressure on the front or back leg. Lean over from the waistline.

Bend your elbow to the side of the body, and extend the elbow, and then bring it back to a bending position.

Rowing

Back – Your front leg is bent and your back leg is straight. Your weight is centered, so there is no pressure on the front or back leg. Lean over from your waistline.

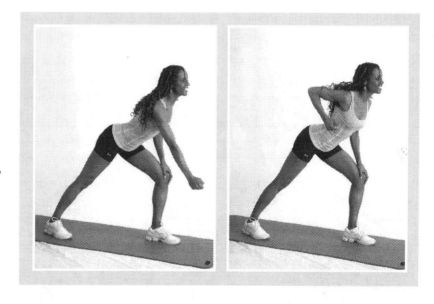

With your left hand on your knee, your right arm rows from the floor as though pulling up weeds. Bend at the elbow and pull, keeping your arms close to your body.

Chapter Two: Basic Exercises

Bicep Curls

Biceps – Stand with your feet hip-width apart, palms facing front and arms extended. Bend your arms at the elbows, and extend back to their original position.

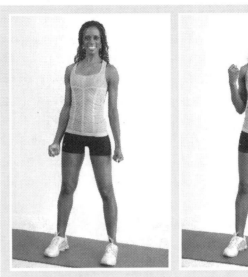
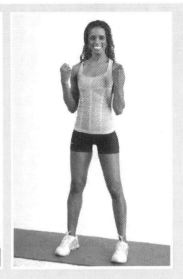

Sit-ups

Abdominals – Sit straight, with your shoulders back and chest out, knees bent and feet flexed, arms shoulder-level, straight in front of you. Roll back (lower back, middle and upper back, head) into a lying position with arms over your head and then roll up (head, upper back, middle, and lower back) to your original position..

Chapter Two: Basic Exercises

Push Ups

Push Ups/Chest – Start on the floor with your hands a little wider than your shoulders, hands straight, with knees on the mat and the tops of the feet on the floor together. Bend at the elbows and extend.

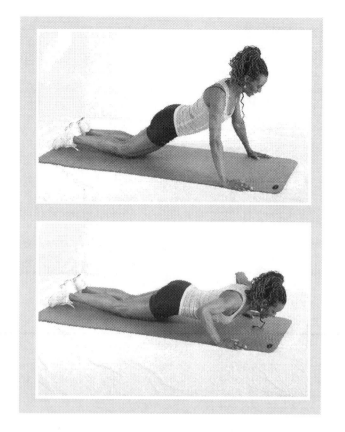

Push Ups Full/ Chest, Core – Start on the floor, arms wider than the shoulders and body extended and straight. Feet two to three inches apart. Bend at the elbow and extend, keeping the rest of the body isolated.

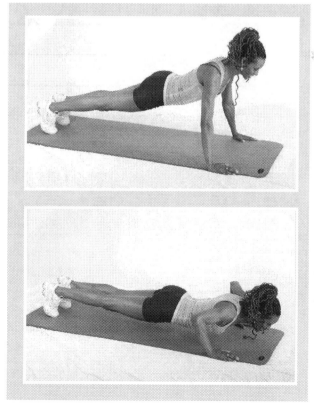

Lateral Side Raise/ Shoulders

Shoulders – Stand with your feet wide and parallel, bring your arms out to each side at shoulder level toward the front of your body. Elbows are soft (not fully extended).

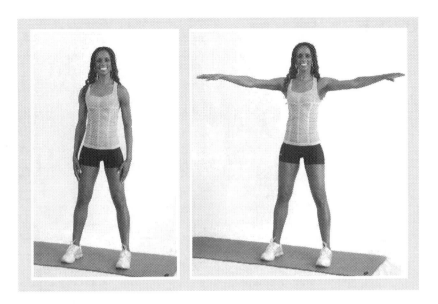

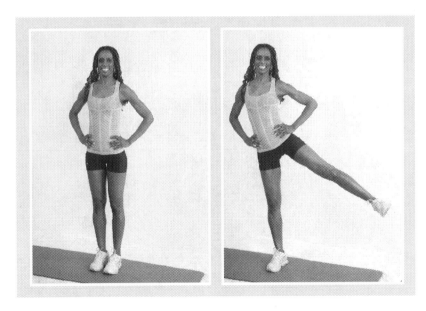

Lateral Side Raise/ Hips

Hips – Standing with both feet together, weight centered, lift your leg in a sweeping motion out to the side with knees toward the front. Change legs.

Chapter Two: Basic Exercises

Leg Raise/Rear

Gluteus Maximus – Standing with both feet together, weight centered, lift your leg (straight) in a sweeping motion behind you, keeping your knees toward the front. Change legs.

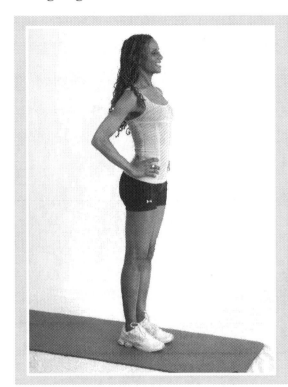
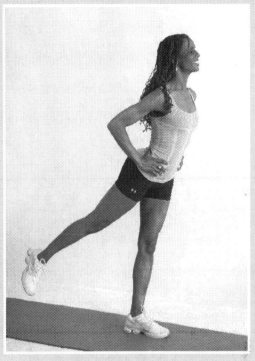

CHAPTER THREE

Functional Focus

Chapter Three: Functional Focus

Functional Focus

The following are exercises to strengthen and tone each muscle group. I hear many say, "I want to tone my arms or my butt, etc." The following exercises show you how to focus on areas of the body, but remember that it is very important to work out the full body for balance. You can, however, put emphasis on targeting certain body parts to achieve the physical goals that you are longing for.

Make sure that you rest thirty to sixty seconds between each exercise. Perform them exactly as demonstrated. For more instruction, get the *"Working Out with Lazet"* DVD. Remember, any time you work out, it is important to warm up first for at least five minutes and to stretch at the end. Always!

What is a warm-up? Marching in place, walking vigorously, running, jumping rope, dancing, biking, *"Working Out with Lazet,"* etc.

Featuring what I call the "functional focus," these exercises, along with stretching at the end, can be performed for the rest of your life. Body building is designed to be performed only for a short time. Functional exercises prepare you for a lifetime of pushing, pulling, twisting, moving, running, jumping, and having fun!

Chapter Three: Functional Focus

Abdominals

Full Abs – Sit straight with your shoulders back and chest out, knees bent and feet flexed. Arms are at shoulder level, extended in front of you. Roll back (lower back, middle, upper, and head) to a lying position with arms overhead and then roll up (head, upper back, middle, and lower) to your original position.

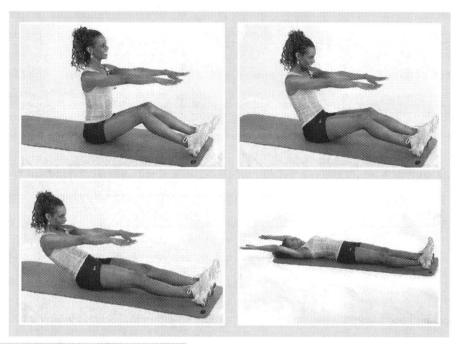

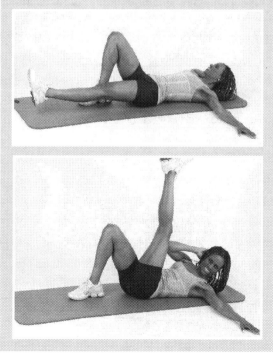

Obliques – Start lying on your back with one knee bent and the other leg straight. The arm opposite the straight leg is behind your head, and other arm is extended to the side, straight out from the shoulder. The extended leg comes up to meet the opposite shoulder. Then move back to the original position.

Chapter Three: Functional Focus

Upper/Lower Crunch – Lie on your back with your knees bent and feet flat on the floor. Arms overhead. Lift upper and lower body, moving arms from over the head to over the knees.

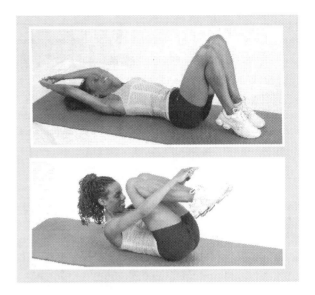

Lower Abs – Lie flat on the mat with both legs extended straight up so that your body forms an L shape. Lower the left leg and then bring it back to the original position. Lower the right leg and then bring it back to the original position. Make sure to keep your lower back pressed into the floor during this exercise.

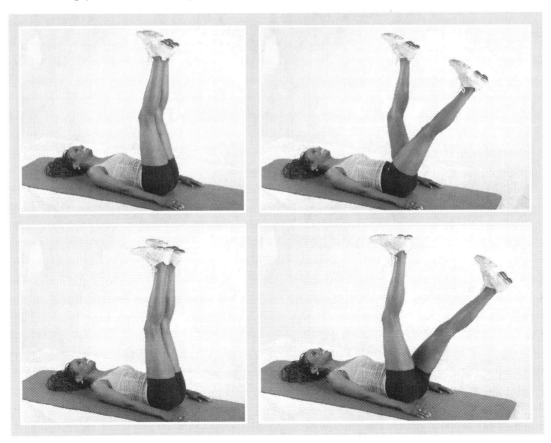

Chapter Three: Functional Focus

Bicycle – Start by lying on your back with your knees to your chest. With hands behind your head and arms flat, chin up, bicycle your legs and twist your upper body, coordinating each arm with the opposite leg.

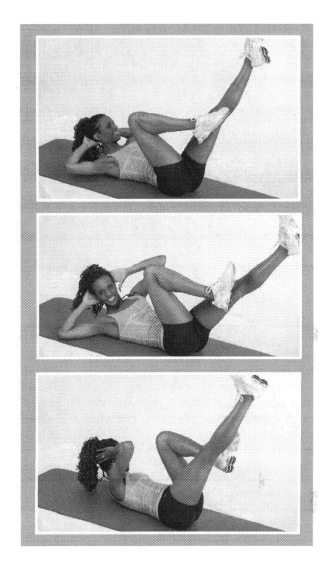

Chapter Three: Functional Focus

Legs

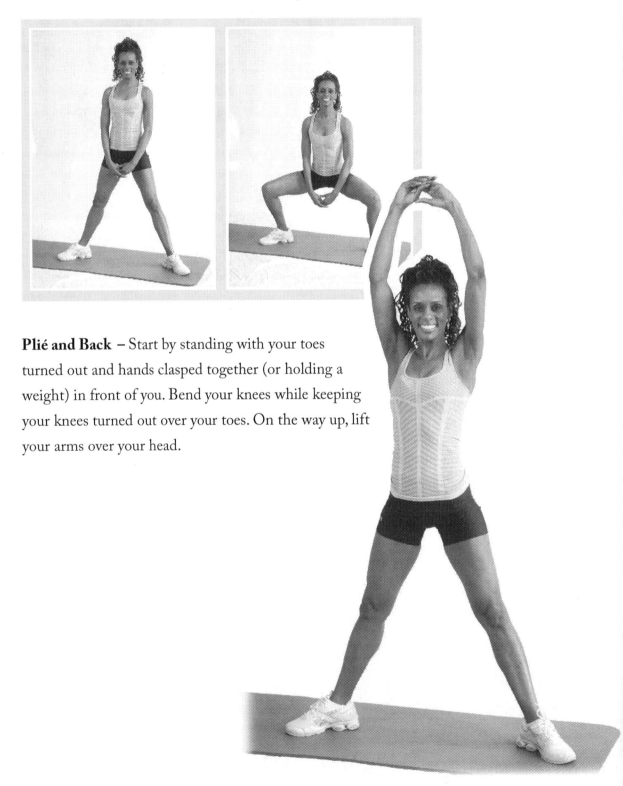

Plié and Back – Start by standing with your toes turned out and hands clasped together (or holding a weight) in front of you. Bend your knees while keeping your knees turned out over your toes. On the way up, lift your arms over your head.

Chapter Three: Functional Focus

Backward Lunge – Start by standing with your feet together. Lift one leg up to hip level and then bring the leg behind you and bend the knee to ninety degrees. Then return to a standing position.

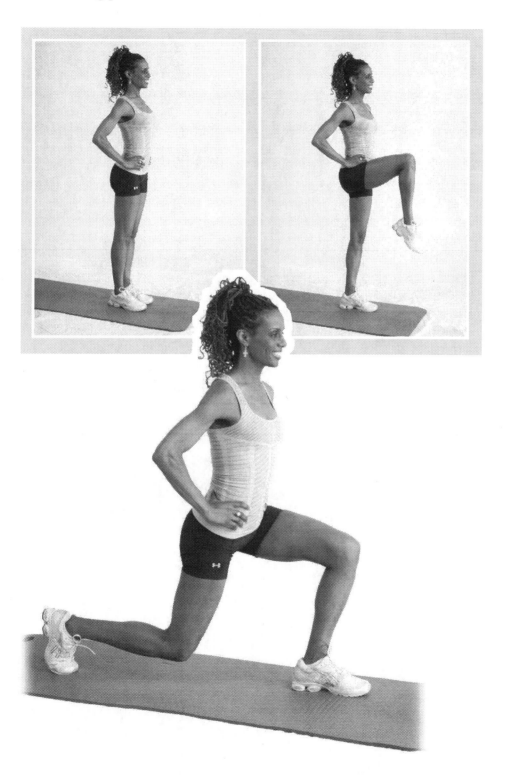

Chapter Three: Functional Focus

Leg Abduction – Start in a standing position with your feet about an inch apart. Lift one leg up to hip level, back down to the center, and then sweep your leg out to the side (hip).

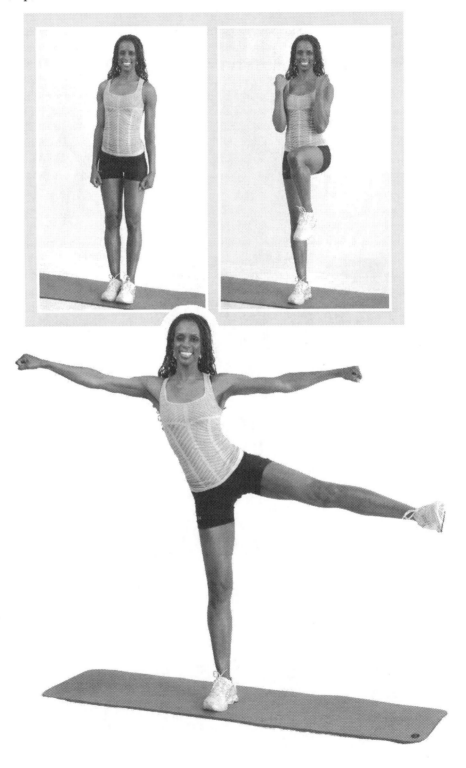

Chapter Three: Functional Focus

Lunge Forward – Start in a standing position with feet hip-width apart. Step forward, bending at the knee to a ninety-degree position where your knee is over the ankle (not over the toes) and then return to the original position.

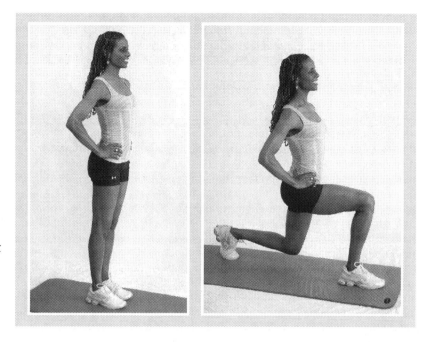

Curtsy – Start in a standing position with feet parallel, about hip-width apart. Bend one leg behind you on a diagonal and then return to the original position.

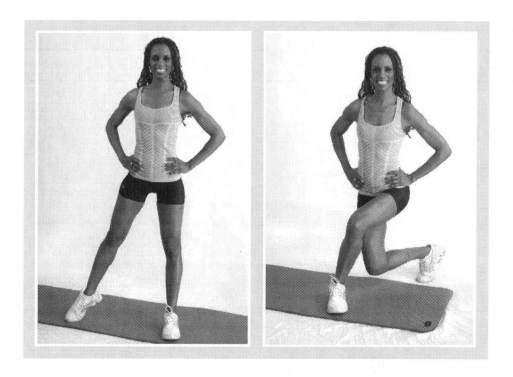

Chapter Three: Functional Focus

Gluteus Maximus (Butt)

Squats – Start with your feet parallel and hip-width apart. Flex your hips and your knees to a ninety-degree angle, keeping your knees over your feet, with arms in front of you, and then return to original position.

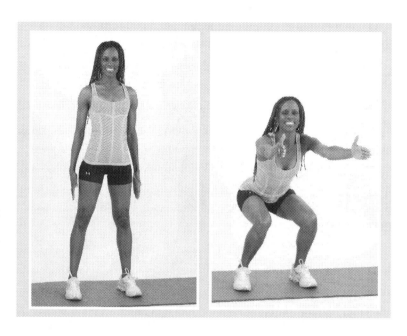

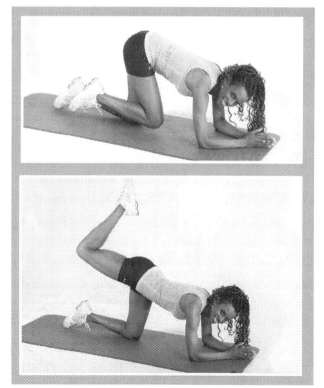

Leg Lifts/Floor – Start on your elbows/forearms and knees, with your body fully balanced on each side. Lift one leg up and back to a ninety-degree angle and return to original position.

Chapter Three: Functional Focus

Hip Abductors – Stand with your feet parallel and hip-width apart. Lift and sweep one leg out to the side, keeping your knees forward, and then back to the original standing position.

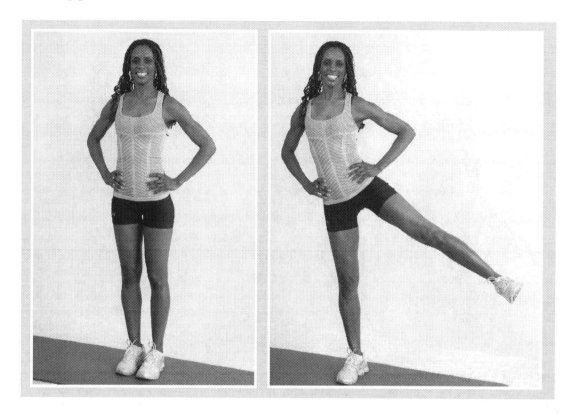

Chapter Three: Functional Focus

Walking Lunges – Start in a standing position with feet parallel. Step forward, bending to a ninety-degree position, and then bring both feet together. Then step forward with the opposite foot to ninety degrees and then back to the original position. This is similar to walking.

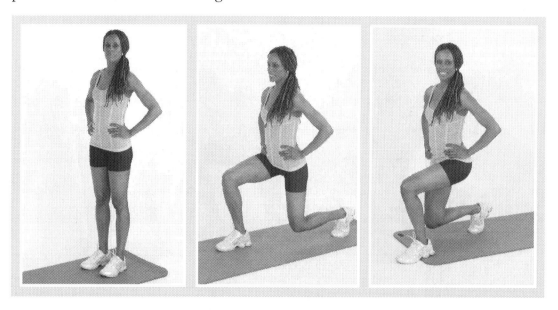

Leg Raise Rear – Standing with both feet together, weight centered, lift the right leg (straight) in a sweeping motion behind you, keeping your knees toward the front. Change legs.

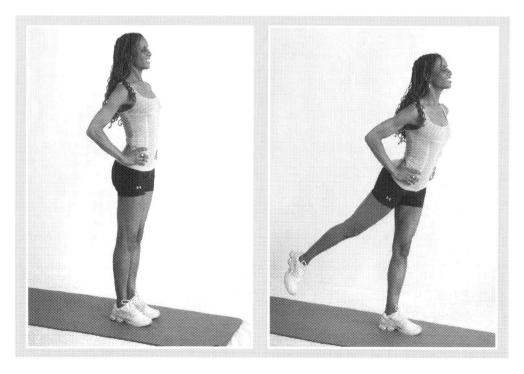

Chapter Three: Functional Focus

Chest

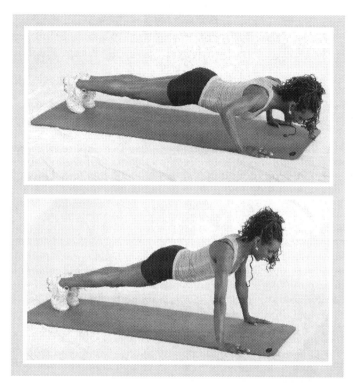

Push-ups Full/ Chest, Core – Start on the floor, arms wider than the shoulders and body extended and straight, feet two to three inches apart. Bend at the elbow and extend, keeping the rest of the body isolated.

Pullovers – Start by lying on your back with your arms over your chest and hands clasped together. Bring your arms over your head and then return them over your chest.

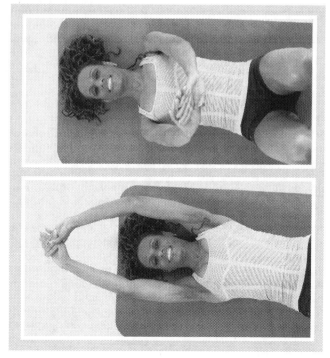

Chapter Three: Functional Focus

Flies – Start by lying on your back with your arms over your chest and rounded as though you are hugging a tree. Open your arms, at shoulder level, and return to your original position.

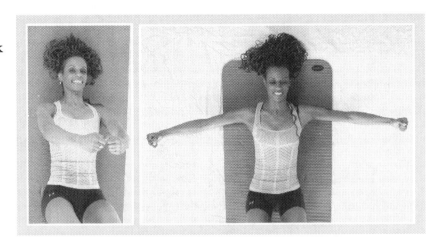

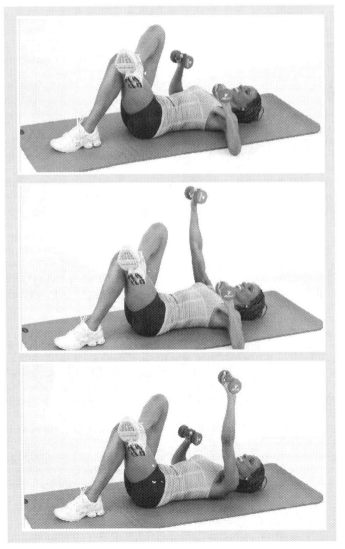

Unilateral Chest – Lying on your back with each arm in a 90-degree position, lift one arm over chest and back and then opposite arm over the chest and back.

Chapter Three: Functional Focus

Shoulders

Overhead Press – Start by standing with your feet shoulder-width apart, arms in a ninety-degree position with stomach in and shoulders back. Push both arms overhead (but do not lock arms) and then back to a ninety-degree position.

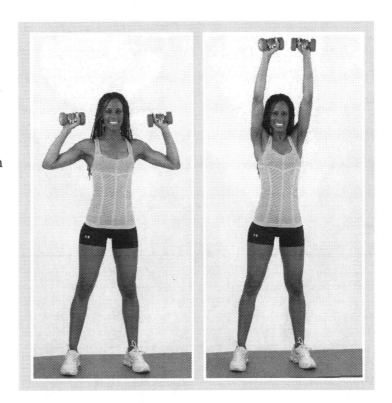

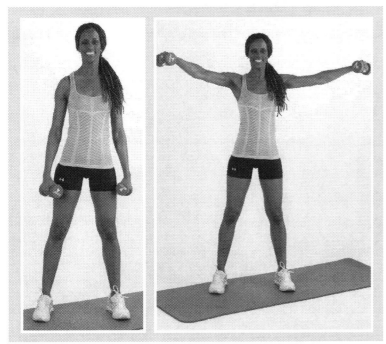

Side Raises – Start by standing with your feet shoulder-width apart, stomach in, shoulders back, arms to your sides. Raise your arms to shoulder level and back to original position.

Chapter Three: Functional Focus

Unilateral Shoulder Press – Start with both arms at a ninety-degree angle. Press your right arm overhead, then come back to a ninety-degree position. Then your left arm overhead and then back to ninety degree position.

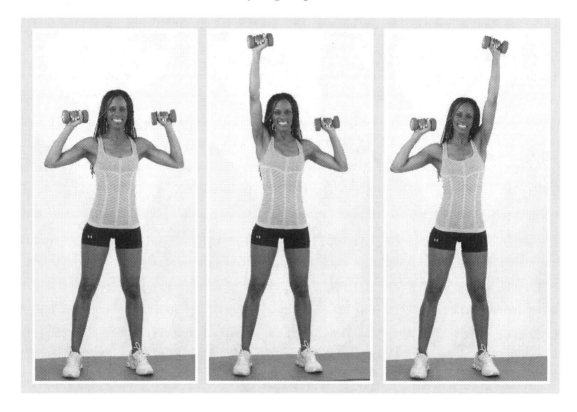

Chapter Three: Functional Focus

Rear Deltoids – Start by standing with your feet shoulder-width apart. You're your knees and lean over from your waistline, keeping your chest out and shoulders back. With arms in front of you and rounded, lift both arms behind you and then back to original position.

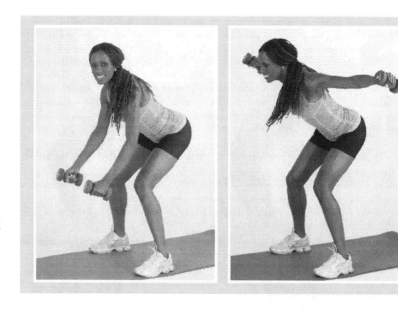

Rear Deltoids/ Rotator – Start by standing with your feet shoulder-width apart, chest out, and shoulders back. Bring the right arm diagonally across the body from the lower left hip over the head. Change arms.

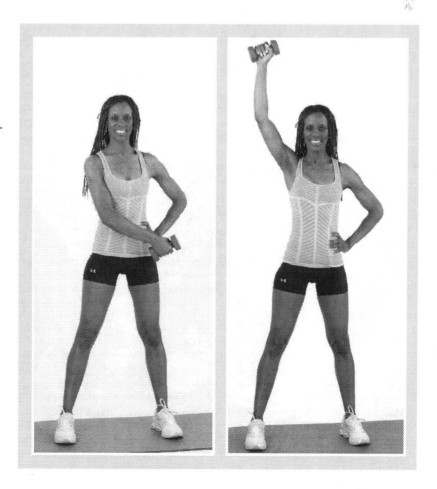

Chapter Three: Functional Focus

Back

Rowing/Unilateral/Upper and Lower – Start with your standing leg bent and your opposite leg lifted behind to hip level and straight. On the same side as the lifted leg, row your arm from an extended position to a flexed position, with chest out and shoulders back. Change position.

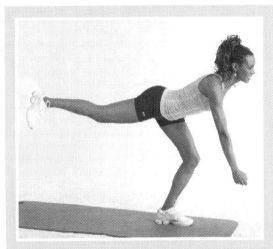
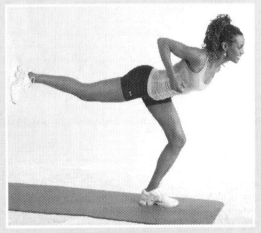

Rowing/Bilateral – Standing with your feet parallel and shoulder-width apart, bend over from your waistline with your chest out and shoulders back. Extend both arms and flex both arms, keeping them close to your body.

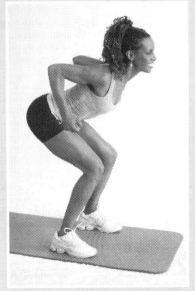
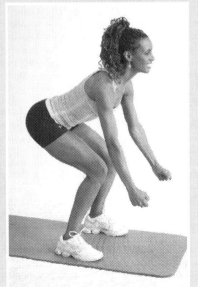

Chapter Three: Functional Focus

Push-up/Back – Start on the floor with your body extended and your arms shoulder-width apart. Keep your hips high, yet level with the rest of the body.

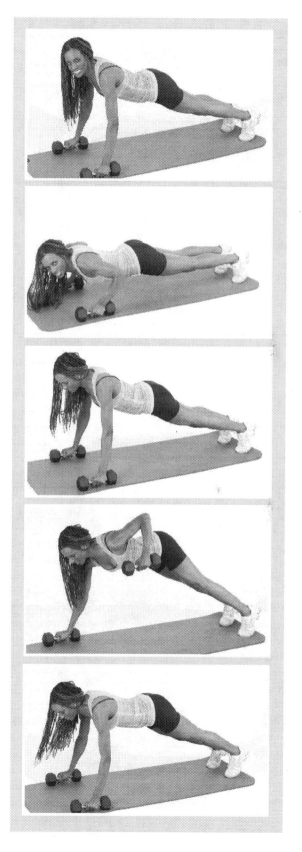

With weights in both hands, bend at the elbow and then extend and row one arm behind and back until it is straight.

Again bend, extend, and lift opposite arm behind, then straight, and back to original position.

Chapter Three: Functional Focus

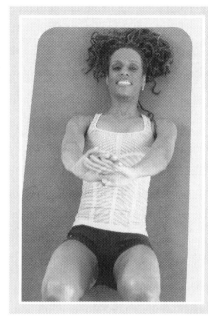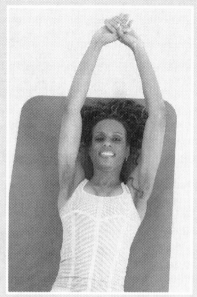

Pullovers – Lie on your back with knees bent and feet flat on the floor. Start with your arms over your chest and rounded as though you are hugging a tree. Extend them over your head and then back over your chest.

Standing Row – Standing in a lunge position, start with your left leg. Lean over from the waistline. With your right arm, row from the floor up, bending your elbow

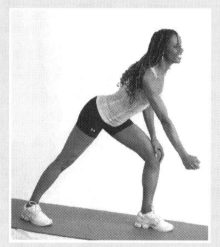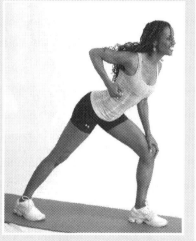

behind you. Change arm and leg.

Chapter Three: Functional Focus

Lower Back –
Lie on your stomach
with your arms
straight overhead.

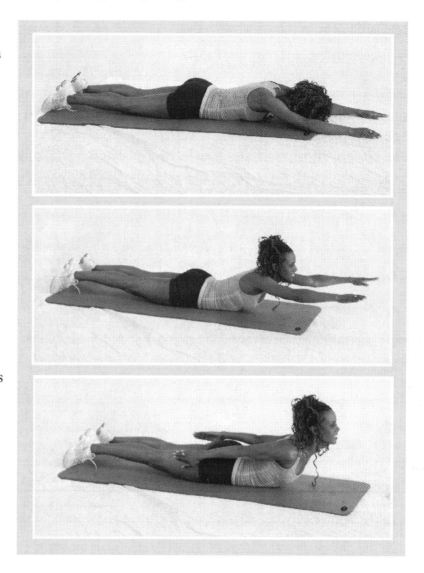

Lift up your chest
and arms and then
move both arms
around the body to
the side of the body,
then move your arms
back around to their
original position.

Chapter Three: Functional Focus

Back and Trunk

(Bonus moves—for those comfortable with the resistance ball)

Lie on your back with your feet centered on the ball.

With your heels, pull the ball toward you.

Then lift your hips up with your feet flat on the ball.

Then bring your hips down.

Roll the ball forward with your heels on the ball to the original position.

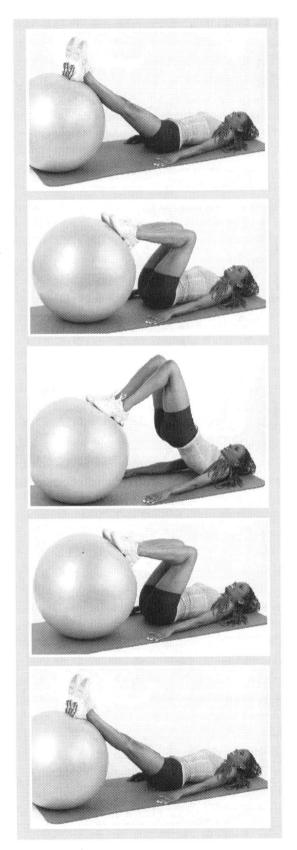

Arms

Tricep Dips – Sit on a chair or bench and place your hands beside your hips with your knees bent and feet flat on the floor. Lift yourself off the chair and extend your arms and then lower yourself, bending your elbows to ninety degrees, and then raise up.

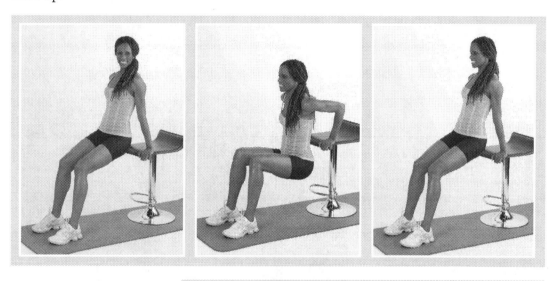

Bicep Curls – Stand with your feet shoulder-width apart and parallel. Start with both arms straight and to your side and then bend your elbows and extend.

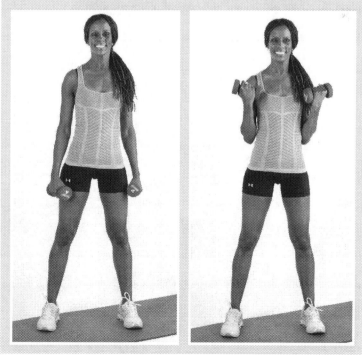

Chapter Three: Functional Focus

Bicep/Shoulder Combo – Start with your feet shoulder-width apart and parallel. Start with both arms to your side, bend, press overhead, bend, and extend back to original position.

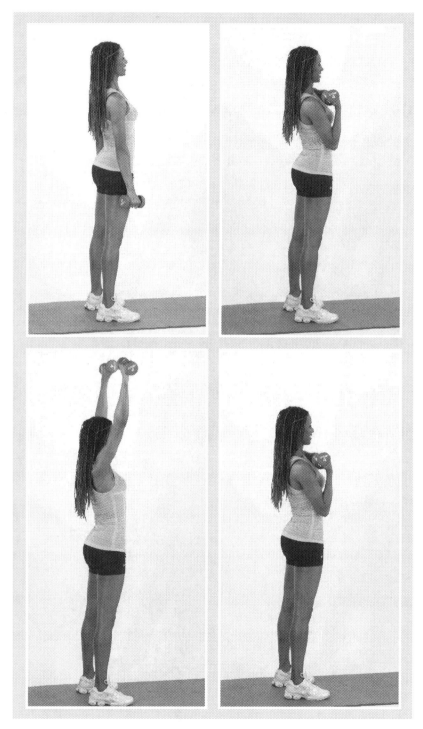

Chapter Three: Functional Focus

Push-ups/Chest – Start on the floor with hands a little wider than the shoulders, hands straight, with knees on the mat and the tops of the feet on the floor together. Bend at the elbows and extend.

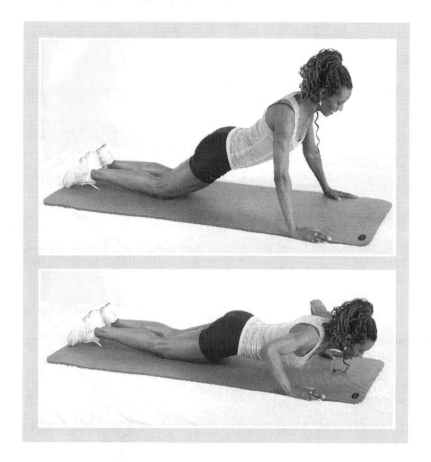

Tricep – Standing in a lunge position, lean over from the waistline. Pull one arm behind you to a bent position. Keep elbow stable and extend. Repeat with other arm.

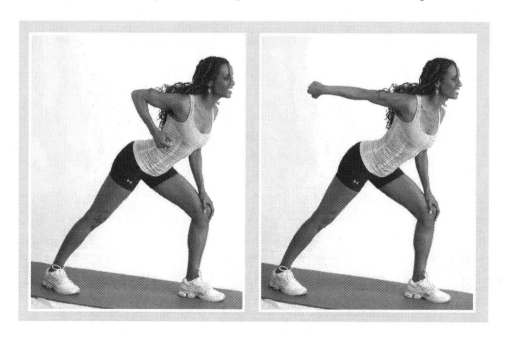

Core

Plank – Lie on the side of your body and pretend you are on a straight line. Your bottom arm is in a ninety-degree position, and the opposite arm is on your hip.

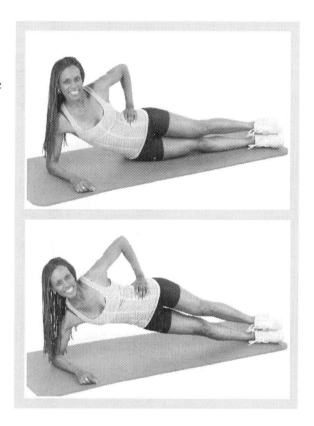

Lift your hip up and then lower it. Change sides.

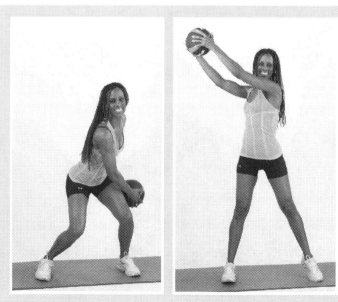

Diagonal Waistline – Start by standing with your feet parallel, hip-width apart. Bend your knees and bring your arms to the left side of your body. With straight arms and straight knees, swing your arms diagonally up to the right side of your body and return to original position. Change sides.

Chapter Three: Functional Focus

Plank on Resistance Ball

(Bonus moves—for those comfortable with the resistance ball)

Lie on your back with your feet centered on the ball.

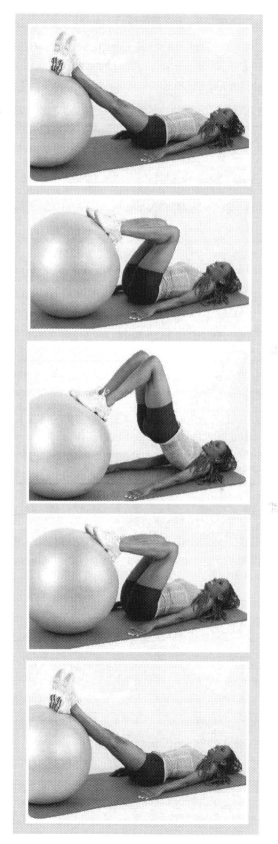

With your heels, pull the ball toward you.

Then lift your hips up with your feet flat on the ball.

Bring your hips down.

Roll the ball forward with your heels to the original position.

Chapter Three: Functional Focus

Abdominals on Resistance Ball
(Bonus moves—for those comfortable with the resistance ball)

Start with arms shoulder-width apart.

With shoelaces on ball, bend your knees with hips high.

Extend your legs and return to your original position.

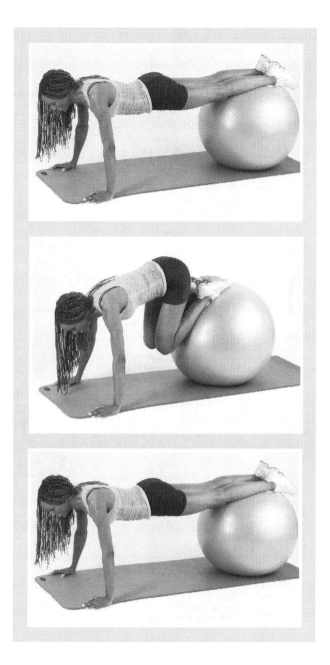

Chapter Three: Functional Focus

Stretch

Lower Back – Start by lying on your back with both knees to your chest. Place your hands right under your knees and squeeze, stretching your lower back.

Then extend one leg and squeeze the other and hold. Repeat with other leg.

Hamstring – Grab your ankle or calf and extend leg over your head.

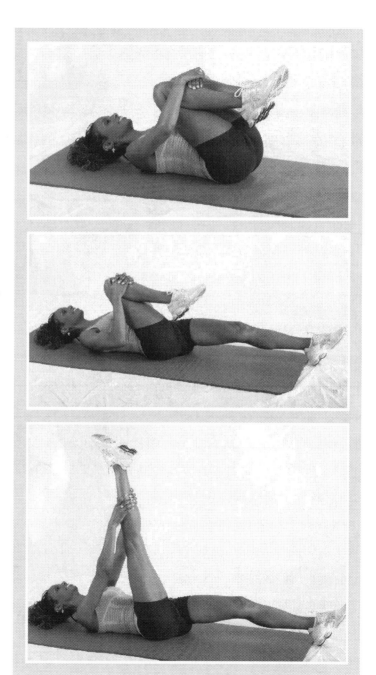

Chapter Three: Functional Focus

Hip and Hamstring – Put both feet flat on the floor.

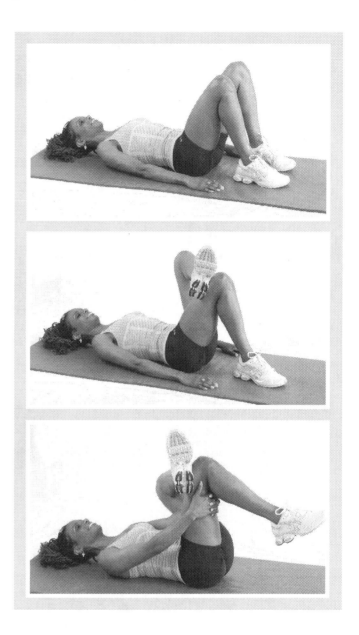

Cross your left leg over your right leg and grab the right thigh.

Pull slightly toward you. Repeat with opposite leg.

Chapter Three: Functional Focus

Waistline, Lower Back, Hips, Arms –Sit up with your knees bent and your ankles crossed. Keep your stomach tight, your chest out, and your shoulders back. With your left arm, reach up overhead and then lean over to the right, keeping your ear over your knee. Lift up your opposite arm and repeat.

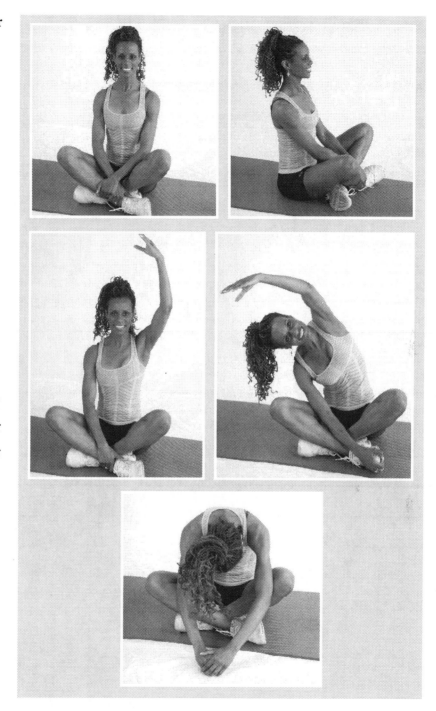

Chapter Three: Functional Focus

Spine, Lower Back, Hamstring, Arms – Place your right leg in front and keep your left leg bent.

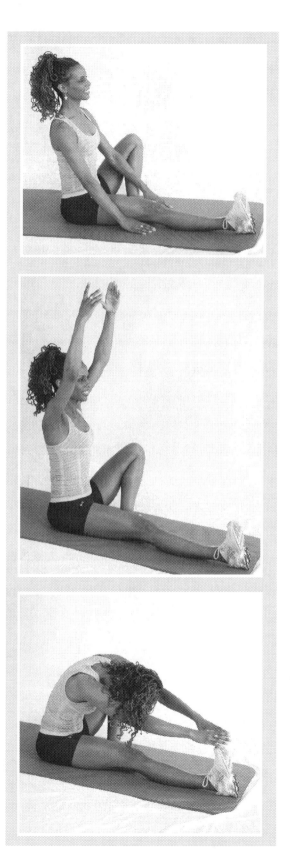

Place both arms over your head and reach forward, grabbing your calf, ankle, or foot.

Bend at the waistline and position your head over your knee. Change legs and repeat.

Chapter Three: Functional Focus

Hamstring, Hips, Waistline, Arms – Straddle your legs with arms shoulder-height out to both sides.

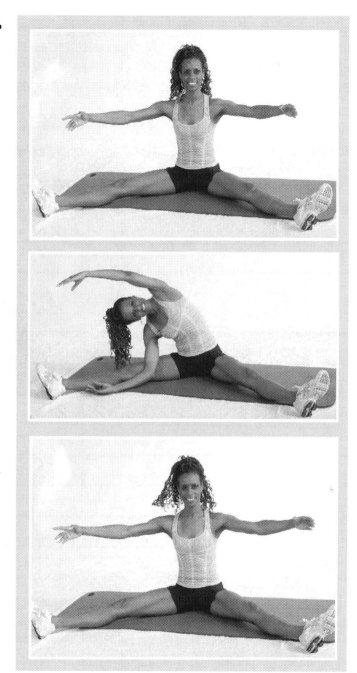

Lift your left arm overhead and bend at the waistline to the right with your ear to your knee.

Lift up slowly and come back to center.

Chapter Three: Functional Focus

Lift right arm overhead and bend at the waistline to the left with ear to the knee.

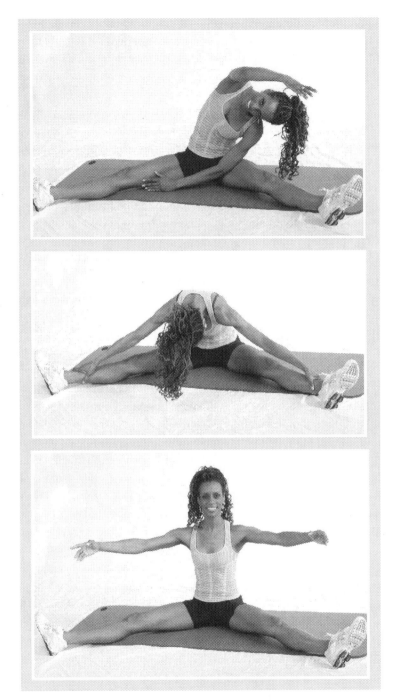

Lean over from the waistline to the center of your straddle with your head toward the floor. Hold your position.

Breathe and then return to the original position.

CHAPTER FOUR

Fifteen Minutes, Fast and Fun

Chapter Four: Fifteen Minutes, Fast and Fun

Fifteen Minutes, Fast and Fun

This is a full-body, fifteen-minute workout for those with a busy lifestyle. Perform this workout every other day. In six to eight weeks, with eating nutritiously, you will notice incredible results. This workout, performed in the following order, is set up to be performed with no rests in between. If you feel challenged, take your time and rest thirty seconds to one minute in between exercises. Eventually you will build up to exercising with no rests in between. By moving quickly, you will experience a combination of cardio and toning/sculpting, which can result in burning more calories. You can perform these exercises with or without weights. Everyone has fifteen minutes … Let's do this! (If you cannot coordinate upper- and lower-body movements, then just perform the lower-body movements.) For the first three weeks, perform only one set. In three to five weeks, add on a second set. In six weeks, perform two to three sets.

For your warm-up, try playing your favorite song (or how about the song "Press" by Lazet Michaels from the *"Pressing Forward to the High Calling"* CD?) and warm up for five minutes. Jog in place, bike, jump rope, dance, etc.

Squat/Bicep Combo –
10-20 reps, 1-3 sets

Start with your feet parallel, hip-width apart, arms to the side. Bend your hips and knees as though you are sitting in a chair. Then extend (stand) and bend your elbows simultaneously for a bicep curl.

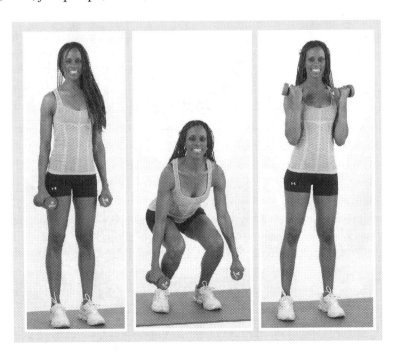

Chapter Four: Fifteen Minutes, Fast and Fun

Row/Tricep Combo – 10-20 reps, 1-3 sets

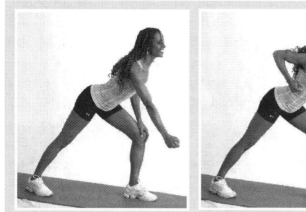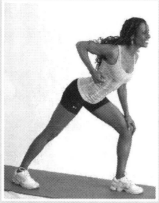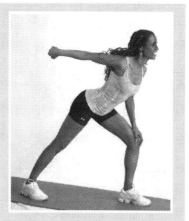

In a lunge position, lean over from your waistline with your chest out and shoulders back. Row from the floor, then bend and extend the elbow, bend again, and return to your original position. Change sides.

Abductor/Core/ Rear Delts – 10-20 reps, 1-3 sets

Start with your feet parallel, hip-width apart. Your right arm is across your left hip. Bend at the knees and sweep your leg out to the side while diagonally sweeping your arm across your body and over your head. Change sides.

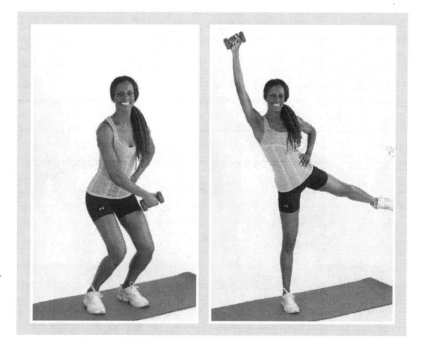

Chapter Four: Fifteen Minutes, Fast and Fun

Push-ups/ Knees Down or Straight – 10-20 reps

Start on the floor with your hands a little wider than your shoulders, hands straight, with your knees on the mat and the tops of your feet on the floor, together. Bend at the elbows and extend.

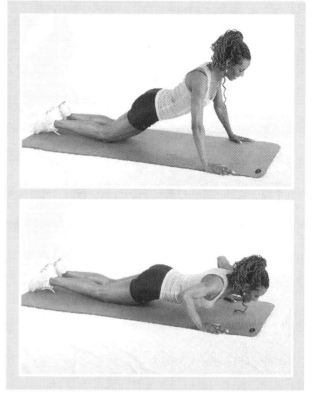

Leg Lifts – 10-30 reps

Start on your elbows/forearms and knees, with your body fully balanced on each side. Lift your leg up and back to a ninety-degree angle and return to the original position.

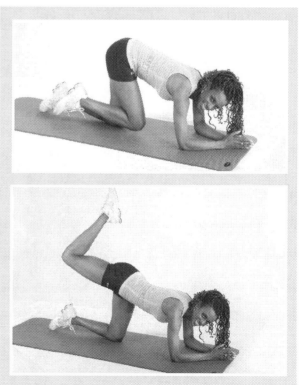

Chapter Four: Fifteen Minutes, Fast and Fun

Full Abs – 8-20 reps

Sit straight, with your shoulders back and chest out, knees bent, and feet flexed. Your arms should be shoulder-level, extended in front of you. Roll back (lower back, middle, upper, and head) to a lying position with arms overhead, and then roll up (head, upper back, middle, and lower) to your original position.

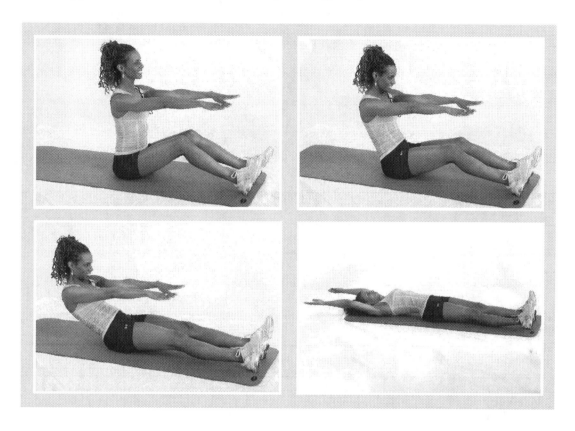

Chapter Four: Fifteen Minutes, Fast and Fun

Upper/Lower Crunch –
8-30 reps

Lie on your back with your knees bent, your feet flat on the floor, and your arms overhead.

Lift your upper and lower body, moving your arms from over your head to over your knees.

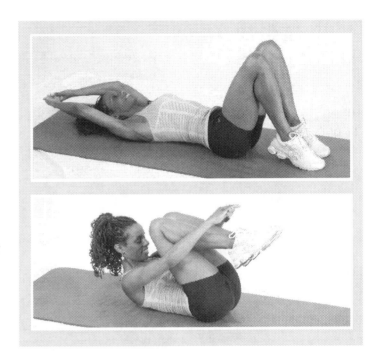

Plank – 6-10 reps

Lie on the side of your body and pretend you are on a straight line. Your bottom arm is in a ninety-degree position, and your opposite arm is on your hip.

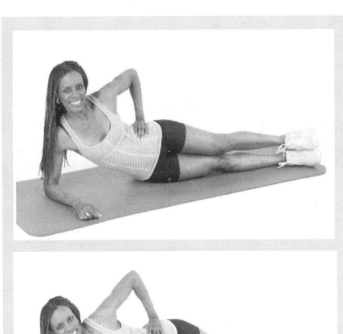

Lift your hip up and then lower it. Change sides.

Stretch—always stretch!
Refer to pages 73-78.

CHAPTER FIVE

Full Workout

Full Workout

This is a full-body workout divided into two days. Day one workout may take forty minutes to one hour, depending on how efficiently you work out. Before doing the full-body workout, remember to warm up for at least five minutes. If you plan on doing a full cardio workout first, it should be at least twenty minutes to one hour. While working out, remember to encourage yourself in the Lord by putting on your favorite ministry podcast, CD, or DVD if you are on a bike or a treadmill. Feed your body and your spirit. God wants to be in the middle of all you do. If you do not care for music or any noise while working out, then pray. Decree and declare … Command your morning! Encourage yourself in the Lord! For example …

Lord, you are great and you do miracles so great … there is no one else like you. I thank you, Lord, that you are healing my mind, my soul, my spirit, my ears, my eyes, my heart, my lungs, my back, my knees, my hips, my ankles, my shoulders, my feet, and my hands. Thank you for the sunshine, thank you for the grass and trees. Thank you for the healing power of oxygen, too. It's healing me. I know that I cannot make it through without you, Lord. But I also know that when I am weak, you are strong, and today this workout is easy and fun because your yoke is easy and your burden is light.

Let's work out and worship!

Day One

Plié & Back – 10-20 reps, 1-3 sets

Start by standing with your toes turned out and hands clasped together (or holding a weight) in front of you. Bend your knees while keeping your knees turned out over your toes. On the way up, lift your arms over your head.

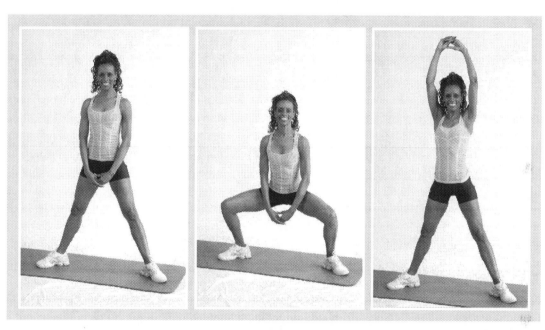

Diagonal Waistline –
10-20 reps, 1-3 sets

Start by standing with your feet parallel, hip-width apart. Bend your knees and bring your arms to the left side of your body. With straight arms and straight knees, swing your arms diagonally up to the right side of your body and return to original position. Change sides.

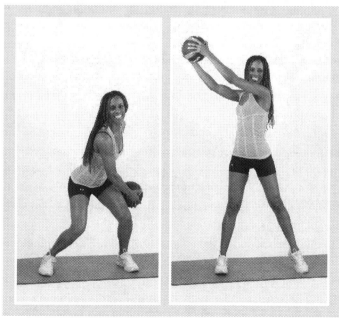

Chapter Five: Full Workout

Squat/Bicep Shoulder Press –

10-20 reps, 1-3 sets

Start by standing with your feet hip-width apart. Bend to ninety degrees. Extend and curl bicep simultaneously. Then shoulder press overhead, back to bicep curl and arms down.

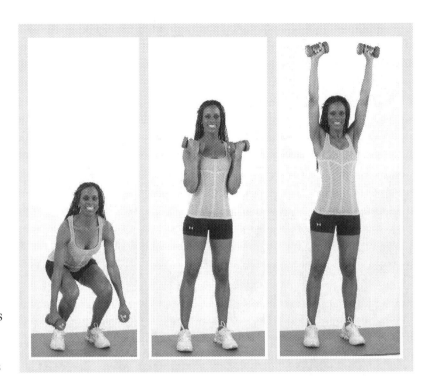

Tricep Dips –

5-20 reps, 1-3 sets

Sit on a chair or bench and place your hands beside your hips with your knees bent and feet flat on the floor. Lift yourself off the chair and extend your arms and then lower yourself, bending your elbows to ninety degrees, and then raise up.

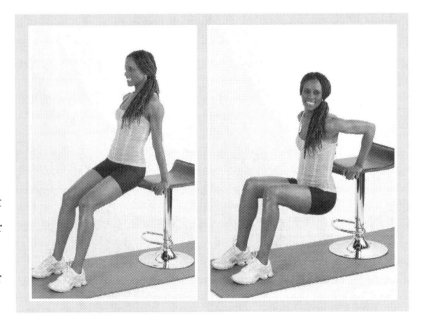

Chapter Five: Full Workout

Lunge/Shoulder Combo – 5-20 reps, 1-3 sets

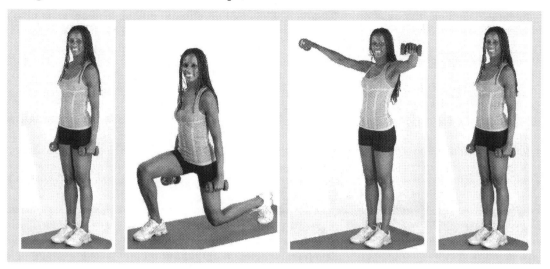

Start by standing with your feet parallel, two to three inches apart. Step forward to a ninety-degree angle in front and back. Come back to a parallel standing position. Lift arms to sides and lower. Change legs.

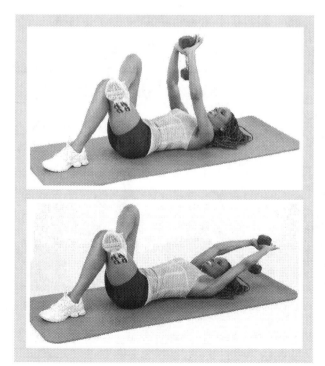

Pullovers – 10-20 reps, 1-3 sets

Lie on your back with your arms over your chest and place both palms under neck of weight.

Bring your arms over your chest and then over your head and return to the original position.

Chapter Five: Full Workout

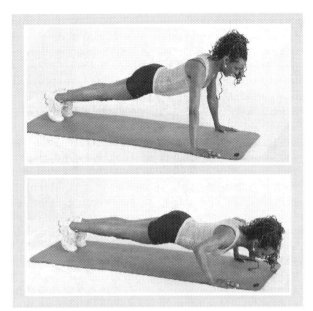

Push Ups – 10-20 reps, 1-3 sets

Start on the floor with hands a little wider than the shoulders, hands straight, with knees on the mat and the tops of the feet on the floor together. Bend at the elbows and extend.

Chest Flies on Resistance Ball

10-20 reps, 1-3 sets.

(Bonus moves—for those comfortable with the resistance ball)

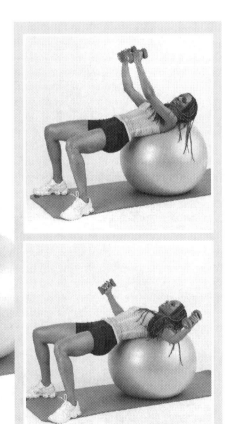

Start in a seated position, sitting in the middle of the ball with feet parallel and a little wider than your hips. Slowly roll your torso forward so that your head and upper back are comfortable on the ball. Push up your hips (which are not on the ball), keeping them high. Start with the weights (your hands) over your chest, with arms rounded. Open your arms to the side while controlling the weights and then bring the weights back together.

Chapter Five: Full Workout

Full Abs – 10-20 reps, 1-3 sets

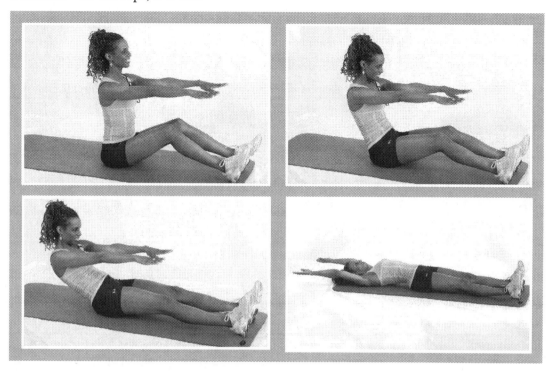

Sit straight with your shoulders back and chest out, knees bent and feet flexed. Your arms should be shoulder-level, extended in front of you. Roll back (lower back, middle, upper, and head) to a lying position with your arms over your head, and then roll up (head, upper back, middle, and lower) to the original position.

Chest Press – 10-20 reps, 1-3 sets

Start by lying on the floor with both knees bent and your feet wider than hip-width or one leg crossed over the other. Start with both arms at ninety degrees.

Lift both weights together over your chest and then return to ninety degrees.

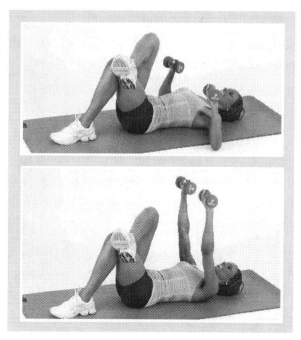

Chapter Five: Full Workout

Obliques – 8-20 reps

Start by lying on your back with one knee bent and the other leg straight. The other arm is extended to the side, straight out from the shoulder.

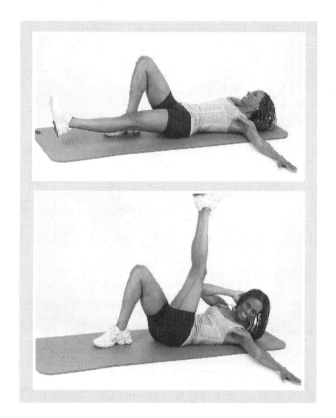

The extended leg comes up and meets the opposite shoulder, then back to your original position.

Upper/Lower Crunch – 10-20 reps

Lie on your back with your knees bent and feet flat on the floor, arms overhead.

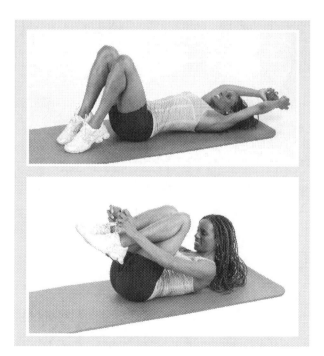

Lift your upper and lower body, moving arms from over the head to over the knees.

Chapter Five: Full Workout

Lower Abs – 5-20 reps

Lie flat on the mat with both legs extended straight up so that your body forms an *L* shape.

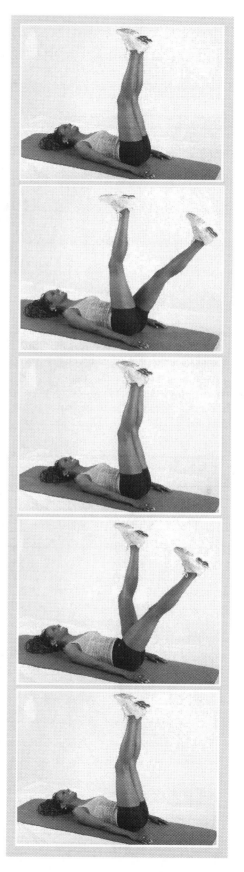

Lower the left leg and then bring it back to the original position.

Lower the right leg and then bring it back to the original position. Make sure to keep your lower back pressed into the floor during this exercise.

Stretch—always stretch!

Refer to pages 73-78.

Chapter Five: Full Workout

Full Workout

Day Two

Rear Deltoids –

5-20 reps, 1-3 sets

Start by standing with your feet shoulder-width apart. Bend your knees and lean over from your waistline, keeping your chest out and shoulders

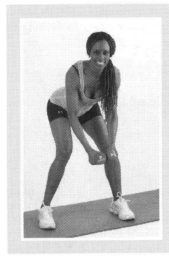
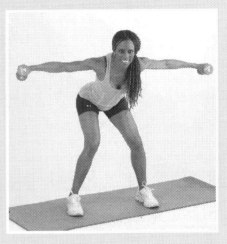

back. With your arms in front of you and rounded, lift both arms behind you and then back to the original position.

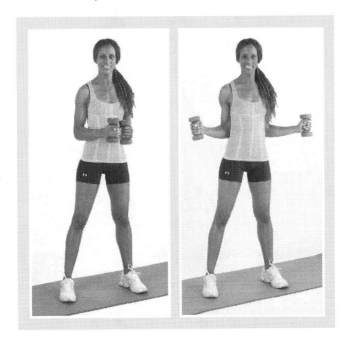

Rotator – 15 reps, 1-3 sets

Start in a standing position with feet parallel, hip-width apart. Bend your arms to ninety degrees and keep your elbows in contact with your waistline as you perform the movement. Start with your hands together, then move them apart, to the sides of the body, and then bring them together again. Bring arms from "in" to "out" for the first set of fifteen and "out" to "in" for the second set of fifteen.

Chapter Five: Full Workout

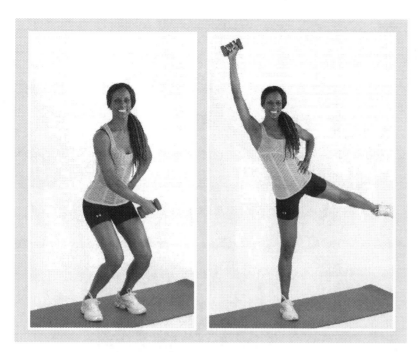

Abductor Leg and Diagonal Arms –

10-20 reps, 1-3 sets

Start with your feet parallel, two to three inches apart. Your right arm is across to your left knee. Raise your left leg and right arm simultaneously. Change leg and arm.

Backward Lunge –

5-20 reps, 1-3 sets

Start by standing with both feet together. Lift one leg up to hip level and then bring the leg behind you and bend the knee to ninety degrees. Then return to a standing position. Change legs.

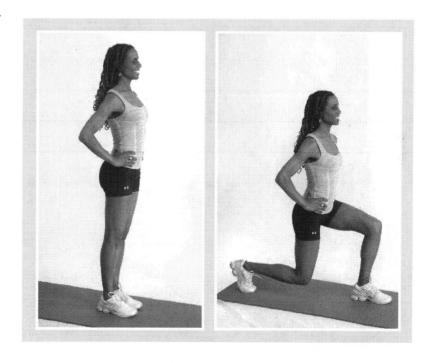

Chapter Five: Full Workout

Leg Lifts – 10-30 reps, 1 set

Start on your elbows/forearms and knees, with body fully balanced on each side. Lift one leg up and back to a ninety-degree angle and return to the original position.

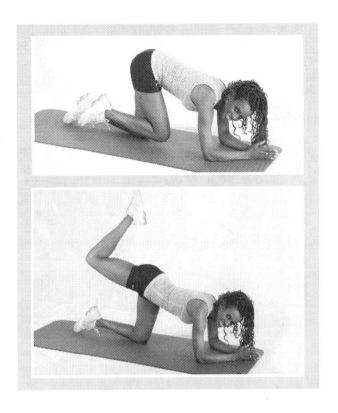

Push-ups/Chest – 10-20 reps, 1-3 sets

Start on the floor, arms wider than the shoulders and body extended and straight, feet two to three inches apart.

Bend at the elbow and extend, keeping the rest of the body isolated.

Chapter Five: Full Workout

Plank on Resistance Ball –

10-20 reps, 1-3 sets

(Bonus moves—for those comfortable with the resistance ball)

Lie on your back with your feet centered on the ball.

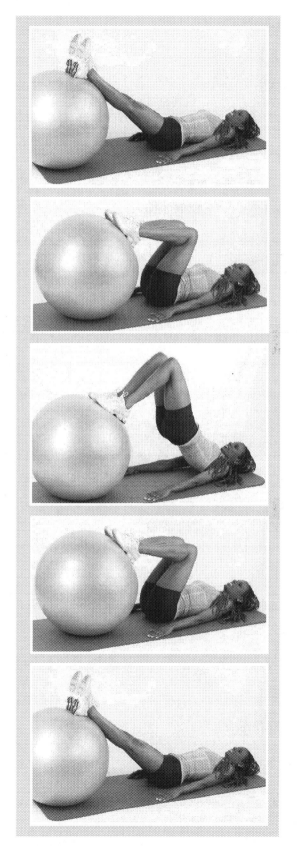

With your heels, pull the ball toward you.

Then lift your hips up with your feet flat on the ball.

Bring your hips down.

Roll the ball forward with your heels to the original position.

Chapter Five: Full Workout

Lower Back –

10-20 reps, 1-3 sets

Lie on your stomach with your arms straight overhead.

Lift up your chest and arms and then move both arms around your body to the side of your body, then move your arms back around to their original position.

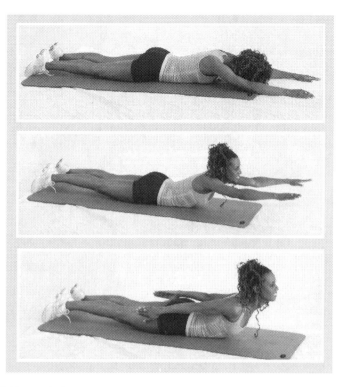

Abdominals on Resistance Ball –

10-20 reps, 2-3 sets
(Bonus moves—for those comfortable with the resistance ball.)

Start with your arms shoulder-width apart. With shoelaces on ball, bend your knees with hips high. Extend your legs and return to the original position.

Full Abs – Refer to page 91.

Stretch—always stretch!
Refer to pages 73-78.

CHAPTER SIX

Devotion and Prayer

Devotion and Prayer

Prayer 1: The Beginning
Weeks 1-4

> *But they that wait upon the Lord shall renew their strength, they shall mount up with wings as eagles, they shall run and not be weary, they shall walk and not faint.*
>
> –Isaiah 40:31

The verse above is a very precious promise to believers. It affirms that God will renew our strength when we need it. When you work out, meditate on this verse, and thank God for all the help that he gives you.

I thank you, Lord that you are the wind beneath my wings. I dare not take on this challenge without you, Lord. I wait upon you, and I believe that you have renewed my strength. I will run and not be weary, and I will walk and not faint. My mind is renewed, my body is renewed, my spirit is renewed, and I am ready for you to change and mold me and make me what you need me to be to walk in your purpose and to walk in your calling. You have made me in your image and in your likeness. I thank you that you have made my body the temple of the holy spirit. Thank you, Lord for the revelation that you live inside me. I am your house, and in my thankfulness I give my body as a living sacrifice in all I do, in all I eat, in all I drink. I work out and worship you, and I work out, and I praise you. For you say that I can do all things through Christ, who strengthens me. Thank you, Lord, that you are my helper. You are my strength. And because of you I am forgetting those things of the past and reaching to what's before … which is life, health, and strength. I am no longer living in laziness, indecision, and double-mindedness. I have decided to press forward and make Jesus my choice. I shall live and not die. I have many days added to my life because of my decision to change. Because of the choices I now make. For Jesus said, *"I am come that*

Chapter Six: Devotion and Prayer

they might have life and that more abundantly" (John 10:10). I do not acknowledge any voices except the voice of God saying, "I wish above all things that you may prosper and be in health" (III John 2). I hear the Holy Spirit say, *"Ask and you shall receive, seek and ye shall find, knock and the doors will be opened unto you." "For I know the plans I have for you,"* declares the Lord, *"plans to prosper you and not to harm you, plans to give you hope and a future"* (Jeremiah 29:11).

Today I pray for the anointing of David. The anointing of praise and worship to come upon me. The anointing to want to dance again, sing again, jump again, leap again, laugh again, play again, and to worship like never before. Today I am excited and expectant of the healing of my mind, of the healing of my body and the healing of my spirit. I will add vegetables and salads and fruit to my diet daily so that I will be filled with the oxygen that you made to heal us. I will plan and stick to my workout schedule and schedule my workout above all other issues of the day. I will think those things that bring forth life, health, and healing; and do those things that bring forth life, health, and healing; and drink and eat those things that bring forth life, health, and healing.

I thank you, Lord, that with you I can do all things, and I am expectant of wholeness and healing in Jesus's name. Amen.

Now remember … no doubt you will hear many voices every morning say, "Oh you don't have to work out today; you can start tomorrow. You don't have to eat right today; it's just one donut." Starting out, schedule three days of the week to work out, and no matter what thoughts come through your mind, say I'm on my way to work out and nothing is going to stop me." Just do it! Get up out of bed, or leave work and just show up. That's more than half of the battle—showing up. If you show up, you will win!

Chapter Six: Devotion and Prayer

Thoughts for the month...

Journal your journey, the highs and the lows, it's all progress that will lead to your goals and your testimony. Journal what you eat, how you feel, your progress mentally, physically and spiritually and your thankfulness.

My Journal – Weeks 1-4

Weight: _____

Body Fat %: _____

Body Mass Index: _____

Measurements: Waist: _____ Chest: _____

    Hips: _____ Arms: _____ Legs: _____

What I eat: _____

_____

_____

_____

How I feel in body, mind and spirit: _____

_____

_____

_____

_____

_____

What I am thankful for: _____

_____

_____

_____

Chapter Six: Devotion and Prayer

Prayer 2
Weeks 4-8

And the Lord God formed man of the dust of the ground, and breathed into his nostrils the breath of life; and man became a living soul.

–Genesis 2:7

God made our bodies in a way that no matter how badly we abuse our bodies, it continues to want to heal. If you break a leg, the blood and oxygen immediately come rushing to the area to start the healing process. The Lord also made the environment (grass and trees and sun) to heal us. If we breathe in … that's God! If we look and acknowledge, we are surrounded by things that heal us. The Lord left the herb-bearing seed for the healing of the nations. God wants us healed and whole. It takes three weeks for our bodies to acclimate to a workout program, and now you are in week four. As you know, you couldn't have made it without the Lord. If you have been consistent, I'm sure that the workout program is much easier for you, and the muscle soreness that you initially experienced should be gone. Strengthening the muscles can initially make you sore, but as the muscles get stronger, the soreness goes away. So let's thank the Lord for his thoughtfulness toward us and ask him to allow us to submit to his healing lifestyle, and in our thankfulness recognize and be in remembrance of all that he has done. Lord, keep us focused and obedient to receive your blessings and we pray …

I thank you, Lord, that I am on my way. I thank you, Lord, that you have given me the encouragement and discipline to make it this far. I thank you, Lord, that I am feeling better. I thank you, Lord, that I am looking better. Never could have made it without you, Lord. Keep me focused, Lord. Keep my mind on you, Lord. Keep my mind on health and healing, Lord. Thank you that my blood is carrying oxygen freely through my veins. Thank you that I will rise above all temptations. Because I Corinthians 10:13 says, *"There hath no temptation taken you but such as is common to man."*

Chapter Six: Devotion and Prayer

Thank you, Lord, that I am encouraging those around me to work out and eat right. Thank you, Lord, that I am empowering my family to work out and eat right. Thank you, Lord, that each week I prepare for the coming week. I grocery shop ahead of time and like the woman in Proverbs 31:14, *"She is like the merchants ships; she bringeth her food from afar."*

I choose only the best food to put into my temple, which is the temple of the Holy Spirit ... the house of God. I take care of the house that the Lord has given me. And I thank you, Lord, because, as I breathe in, I am reminded of the goodness of you. And each time that I breathe in, I experience divine revelation that you are living inside me. And when I eat the healing foods that you created for me, I savor them and crave them. The healing foods and herbs that you have left on this earth for us, give life. Thank you, Lord, that I am getting stronger and better and happier. She girdeth her loins with strength, and strengtheneth her arms. The Proverbs 31 woman works out. David was a warrior, a soldier in the army of the Lord. A soldier has to be disciplined, a soldier has to train, a soldier has to be consistent. David could not do it on his own, but with the help of the Lord he was a warrior and a winner. I imitate the Proverbs 31 woman, and I am reminded that I am a soldier in the army of the Lord! The army works out in preparation to win. And in the end, we win in Jesus's name. Amen.

Chapter Six: Devotion and Prayer

Thoughts for the month...

Journal your journey, the highs and the lows, it's all progress that will lead to your goals and your testimony. Journal what you eat, how you feel, your progress mentally, physically and spiritually and your thankfulness.

My Journal – Weeks 4-8

Weight: _____

Body Fat %:_____

Body Mass Index: _____

Measurements: Waist:_____ Chest:_____

    Hips:_____ Arms:_____ Legs:_____

What I eat: _____

_____

_____

_____

How I feel in body, mind and spirit:_____

_____

_____

_____

_____

_____

What I am thankful for:_____

_____

_____

_____

Chapter Six: Devotion and Prayer

Prayer 3
Weeks 8-12

> *The hand of the Lord was upon me, and he brought me out by the spirit of the Lord and set me in the middle of a valley; it was full of bones. He led me back and forth among them, and I saw a great many bones on the floor of the valley, bones that were very dry. He asked me, "Son of man, can these bones live?" I said, "O Sovereign Lord, you alone know." Then he said to me, "Prophesy to these bones and say to them, 'Dry bones, hear the word of the Lord! This is what the Sovereign Lord says to these bones: I will make breath enter you, and you will come to life."*
>
> –Ezekiel 37:1–7

A sedentary lifestyle can cause you to feel very down and out and bored with life, which I describe as a dry-bone existence. Also, not working out can cause osteoporosis, which makes your bones very dry and brittle and easy to break. Now that you are in your eighth week, do you feel like the moment in Ezekiel where God has breathed his breath in you and you are starting to live again? Now you laugh again (caused by endorphins when you do vigorous exercise) and, without even recognizing it, your bone density is getting stronger every day. We have great reason to offer praise and thanksgiving, and we pray …

I thank you, Lord, for your encouragement again, because I cannot do this without you. Isaiah 40:31 says, *"But they that wait upon the Lord shall renew their strength; they shall mount up with wings as eagles; they shall run, and not be weary, and they shall walk, and not faint."*

Thank you, Lord, that I am walking and not fainting. Thank you, Lord, that my strength is renewed. I thank you, Lord, that I am encouraged by your word, for it is a lamp to my feet and a light to my path. I can do all things through Christ, who strengtheneth me!

Chapter Six: Devotion and Prayer

With each step I take I say, I can do all things through Christ, who strengthens me. As I change the way that I eat … as I make healthier food choices, I say, I can do all things through Christ who strengthens me. As I turn down sodas and sugars and saturated fats, potato chips, fast food, and the like, I say, I can do all things through Christ, who strengthens me. When I get up in the morning tired or get off work and something tells me, "Oh, stay in bed or just go home, you can work out tomorrow," I say I'm working out today because I can do all things through Christ, who strengthens me! I thank you, Lord, that I decree and declare that I am healthy, happy, and whole. I thank you, Lord, that the gift of health and healing comes along with life, laughter, joy, and peace. As I work out, I think of your goodness, canceling out stress, depression, hurt, and pains of the past, any unwillingness to forgive, any bitterness, any offenses. I stamp out any thought that is not like you.

I put encouraging word tapes in my head while I work out, music that reminds me of your goodness and greatness, for you are the great I AM. My bones are getting stronger, and I put resistance to them. I no longer walk around with dry-bone mentality and attitude. For the Lord says to prophesy to these dry bones, and he will give them life. I prophesy that I am strong, I am motivated, I am encouraged, I prophesy that the arteries of my heart, brain, and major organs are now washed free of plaque and cholesterol; I am free from the risk of stroke, hardening of the arteries, blindness, hypertension, renal failure, heart attack, angina, and chronic chest pain. I am happy and healthy and ready to be used by you, Lord. Keep me in your will, and keep me in your way. In Jesus's name. Amen.

Chapter Six: Devotion and Prayer

Thoughts for the month...

Journal your journey, the highs and the lows, it's all progress that will lead to your goals and your testimony. Journal what you eat, how you feel, your progress mentally, physically and spiritually and your thankfulness.

My Journal — Weeks 8-12

Weight: _____

Body Fat %:_____

Body Mass Index: _____

Measurements: Waist:_____ Chest:_____

    Hips:_____ Arms:_____ Legs:_____

What I eat: _____

_____

_____

_____

How I feel in body, mind and spirit:_____

_____

_____

_____

_____

_____

What I am thankful for:_____

_____

_____

_____

Chapter Six: Devotion and Prayer

Prayer 4
Weeks 12-16

For the Joy of the Lord is your Strength.

–Nehemiah 8:10

Resistance from working out, whether it is with our natural body weight or with iron, is making us stronger every day. We are able to climb stairs better, walk or run longer distances, lift heavier objects, and push and pull and reach. These small improvements, after twelve weeks, represent God doing his work. The Bible says that physical strength profits little, so we must remember that God is a god of balance. Physical strength is not all that we need. Studying God's way, recognizing him, praising him, and being thankful for what he is doing as we work out, is joyful. And joy is a gladness deep from within. Yes, Lord, thank you that the joy of the Lord is truly our strength! And we pray …

Thank you, Lord, that I have made it this far. Ninety days of walking in health and healing. Thank you, Lord, that you are my joy, the lifter-up of my hands and the lifter-up of my head. Thank you, Lord, that you are my strength. You make me strong. In you I am a warrior, I am stable. No weapon formed against me shall prosper. It won't work. I am working out and making adjustments to my diet to complement who I am in Christ Jesus. I am a high priest, a holy nation, a peculiar people, and it is my time to show forth the praises of him who brought me out of the darkness and into his marvelous light. Look where you brought me in just ninety days. I am excited about what you are doing in my life, Lord. This is only the beginning. And I am going to win this race for a lifetime. My first goal is one year of consistency in the word in my workout and in eating nutritiously. Jehovah Shammah, you are with me and you supply all my needs. You are more than enough for me! Keep me, Lord, in your will and in your way. Keep me, Lord! I decree and declare that I am healed of terminal

Chapter Six: Devotion and Prayer

cancer and tumors, AIDS, seizures, strokes, Parkinson's disease, multiple sclerosis, ALS, emphysema, and sickle cell disease. Psalm 118:17 says, *"I shall not die but live to declare your works in Jesus's name."* Amen.

Chapter Six: Devotion and Prayer

Thoughts for the month...

Journal your journey, the highs and the lows, it's all progress that will lead to your goals and your testimony. Journal what you eat, how you feel, your progress mentally, physically and spiritually and your thankfulness.

My Journal – Weeks 12-16

Weight: _____

Body Fat %:_____

Body Mass Index: _____

Measurements: Waist:_____ Chest:_____

    Hips:_____ Arms:_____ Legs:_____

What I eat: _____

_____

_____

_____

How I feel in body, mind and spirit:_____

_____

_____

_____

_____

_____

What I am thankful for: _____

_____

_____

_____

Chapter Six: Devotion and Prayer

Prayer 5
Weeks 16-20

> *And whatsoever ye shall ask in my name, that will I do, that the Father may be glorified in the son.*
>
> –John 14:13

As we pray for strength, health, healing, focus, and consistency, just know that if you know Jesus Christ as your savior, the Bible says that God will answer your prayer so that the Father may be glorified. Jesus sits on the right hand of God in intercessory prayer for us. So know that you have a prayer partner and that the Lord will deliver you. Stay encouraged; your breakthrough is coming. Your healthy goals are accomplished in Jesus's name. Just continue to walk or run toward your victory! Lord, today we are reminded:

Jesus! Thank you for all you've done for me. I'm stronger and I'm wiser and I'm better—so much better! And it's all because of Jesus. Walk with me, Lord, talk with me, Lord, move with me, Lord, bless me to hear you clearly, Lord. You are my God, and there is no one greater. You are the great I AM. I can do nothing without you, but with you I can do all things in the holy name of Jesus! I thank you that I am healthy, I am healed, and I am whole.

I am renewed, I am restored, I am delivered, I am walking in my purpose because of the holy name of Jesus. I am walking in my destiny because of the holy name of Jesus. Because of the holy name of Jesus, I am who I am today and getting better. I have mental clarity, I have balance; I am an encourager and a motivator and a leader. I spread the good news of the gospel of Jesus Christ, and I spread the good news of health and healing. My new level of health is an example wherever I go. I keep my hand on the plow, and I am holding on to life, for he says that I AM come that they may have life and that more abundantly. I thank you, Lord, for an abundant life. More

Chapter Six: Devotion and Prayer

than enough, overflow. I thank you, Lord, for consistency in the spirit. For you said that a double-minded man should not think that he should get anything from the Lord. I thank you, Lord, that I am consistent with my workout and that I am living a healthy lifestyle, and if I fall off, I quickly come back to you and health. I thank you, Lord, for focus, drive, being rooted and planted and grounded in what is best for me and in what is healing me and in what brings me life! I press forward to the high calling of God in Christ Jesus! In Jesus's name. Amen.

Chapter Six: Devotion and Prayer

Thoughts for the month...

Journal your journey, the highs and the lows, it's all progress that will lead to your goals and your testimony. Journal what you eat, how you feel, your progress mentally, physically and spiritually and your thankfulness.

My Journal – Weeks 16-20

Weight:_____

Body Fat %:_____

Body Mass Index:_____

Measurements: Waist:_____ Chest:_____

   Hips:_____ Arms:_____ Legs:_____

What I eat:_____

_____

_____

_____

How I feel in body, mind and spirit:_____

_____

_____

_____

_____

_____

What I am thankful for:_____

_____

_____

_____

Chapter Six: Devotion and Prayer

Prayer 6
Weeks 20-24

> *Ye shall not need to fight in this battle: set yourselves, stand ye still, and see the salvation of the Lord with you, O Judah and Jerusalem: fear not, nor be dismayed; tomorrow go out against them: for the Lord will be with you.*
>
> –II Chronicles 20:17

You are now almost halfway to the yearly goal of working out and eating nutritiously. Just know that the battle is not yours, but the Lord's! All you have to do is cast your cares on him and show up. You've got the victory! And let's thank the Lord for all that he has done and is doing right now and all that he is going to do for you in the future!

I thank you, Lord, that you said that the battle is not mine but the Lord's. I thank you, Lord, that you have great plans for me—to prosper me and to give me a hope and a future. I say with the hymn writer that my hope is built on nothing less than Jesus's blood and his righteousness. On Christ, the solid rock, I stand. All other ground is sinking sand. I thank you, Lord, that you wish the best for me and that you are sitting on the right hand of God in intercessory prayer for me. I have won the battle in Jesus's name. His yoke is easy, and his burden is light. I decree and declare that the issues that once plagued me are now a thing of the past. I have found a way of eating that is good for me, and the Lord is keeping me. I have found a workout routine that is perfect for me, and it feels good. I feel great. I am growing in you, Lord, for you are the vine, and I am the branches. The battle is not mine but the Lord's. I am winning and I have won and I am encouraged. Working out is fun, and I am going to work out and live a healthy lifestyle for the rest of my life. Amen.

Chapter Six: Devotion and Prayer

Thoughts for the month...

Journal your journey, the highs and the lows, it's all progress that will lead to your goals and your testimony. Journal what you eat, how you feel, your progress mentally, physically and spiritually and your thankfulness.

My Journal — Weeks 20-24

Weight: _____

Body Fat %: _____

Body Mass Index: _____

Measurements: Waist: _____ Chest: _____

    Hips: _____ Arms: _____ Legs: _____

What I eat: _____

_____

_____

_____

How I feel in body, mind and spirit: _____

_____

_____

_____

_____

_____

What I am thankful for: _____

_____

_____

_____

Chapter Six: Devotion and Prayer

Prayer 7
Weeks 24-28

> *What? Know ye not that your body is the temple of the Holy Ghost which is in you, which ye have of God, and ye are not your own? For ye are bought with a price; therefore glorify God in your body, and in your spirit, which are God's.*
>
> –I Corinthians 6:19–20

Thank you, Lord, for the revelation, the knowledge, that the spirit that raised Jesus from the dead now lives inside of me. As I work out and worship, I thank you for the revelation that my body is the temple of the Holy Spirit !

Thank you, Lord, that I have made it more than halfway through the year of walking in health and healing. I am healed in Jesus's name. I glorify you in my body and in my spirit. I glorify your name in all the earth. I magnify you in my body and in my spirit. You are great, and you do miracles so great; there is no one else like you.

As I work out, I am in remembrance of you. For you are my strength, my sword, my shield, my defense. You are the burden-bearer and the heavy-load carrier. I lay all my weights, circumstances, situations, hopes and dreams and vision all on you. For you are making and conforming me into what you want me to be physically, mentally, and spiritually. You are the potter, and I am the clay. I can now see the vision of the best me come into fruition, as you shape me and mold me and make me and break me. I thank you that you have put me back together again. I thank you for the body that you have given me. You have made me an original, and there is no one else like me. No one can do what I do. No one can be who I am. Yes, I thank you for divine revelation that I am the temple of the Holy Spirit. God is in me. God lives in me. God is housed in me. For I am not my own; I was bought with a price. I am redeemed, and I will say so. As I eat, I am in remembrance of you. As I sleep, I am in remembrance of you.

Chapter Six: Devotion and Prayer

For I am not alone. You are here with me. Jehovah Shammah, you are with me, and you supply all my needs. You're more than enough, more than enough for me.

My bones are stronger in Jesus's name. My hips are stronger in Jesus's name. My knees are healed and stronger in Jesus's name. My shoulders are stronger in Jesus's name. My core and my frame are stronger in Jesus's name. I am girded as a soldier in the army of the Lord. I am flexible in Jesus's name. I thank you, Lord, that I am healed and that I am whole. In Jesus's name. Amen.

Chapter Six: Devotion and Prayer

Thoughts for the month...

Journal your journey, the highs and the lows, it's all progress that will lead to your goals and your testimony. Journal what you eat, how you feel, your progress mentally, physically and spiritually and your thankfulness.

My Journal – Weeks 24-28

Weight: _____

Body Fat %:_____

Body Mass Index: _____

Measurements: Waist:_____ Chest:_____

    Hips:_____ Arms:_____ Legs:_____

What I eat: _____

_____

_____

_____

How I feel in body, mind and spirit:_____

_____

_____

_____

_____

What I am thankful for:_____

_____

_____

_____

Chapter Six: Devotion and Prayer

Prayer 8
Weeks 28-32

"But for you who revere my name, the sun of righteousness will rise with healing in its wings. And you will go out and leap like calves released from the stall. Then you will trample down the wicked; they will be ashes under the soles of your feet on the day when I do these things," says the Lord Almighty.

–Malachi 4:2/ NIV

Thank you, Lord, that in you we are alive, energetic, and more than conquerors. In you, we always win! And I thank you …

Thank you, Lord, that "No weapon formed against me shall prosper." Thank you Lord for your healing, wonder-working power. I am healed from the tip of my head to the soles of my feet. And I pray.

I thank you, Lord, that your desire for me is to run and jump and leap out of the stall and to trample down the wicked and for the wicked to be under the soles of my feet. I am no longer weak; I am strong, and I envision myself as you see me, Lord. I am a soldier in the army of the Lord, wearing the breastplate of righteousness, carrying the shield of faith, the sword of the spirit, and my feet are shod with the gospel of peace. I wait upon you, Lord, for the battle is not mine but the Lord's. I see my healing in the practical ways of life. I see my healing daily. I see miracles daily. You woke me up this morning and started me on my way. You put the thought of wanting to be whole again in my mind. You give us the opportunity to choose life or death, and I choose life! I was dead in my sins and dead in my attitude, living a dry-bone life, and now you have made me whole again. Now I experience peace in my body, peace in my mind, peace in my spirit. No more confusion, no more stress, no more depression, no more overeating; I no longer eat the foods that kill me but the foods that bring me life. Foods that are full of vitamins and herbs. I love to move and walk and run and

Chapter Six: Devotion and Prayer

go and play with my children and laugh and sing and worship and praise and dance like David danced. I am a champion in Jesus's name. I am a winner in Jesus's name. I am an example for all to see. Living a healthy lifestyle is my ministry. The battle is not mine but the Lord's, and my foot is on the enemy's neck. I tread upon serpents and scorpions and over all the evils of this world. With my faith I shield myself from Satan's fiery darts. Greater is he that is in me than he that is in the world. I am a winner today in Jesus's name! Amen.

Chapter Six: Devotion and Prayer

Thoughts for the month...

Journal your journey, the highs and the lows, it's all progress that will lead to your goals and your testimony. Journal what you eat, how you feel, your progress mentally, physically and spiritually and your thankfulness.

My Journal — Weeks 28-32

Weight: _____

Body Fat %: _____

Body Mass Index: _____

Measurements: Waist:_____ Chest:_____

    Hips:_____ Arms:_____ Legs:_____

What I eat: _____

_____

_____

_____

How I feel in body, mind and spirit:_____

_____

_____

_____

_____

_____

What I am thankful for:_____

_____

_____

_____

Chapter Six: Devotion and Prayer

Prayer 9
Weeks 32-36

> *Do you not know that in a race all the runners run, but only one gets the prize? Run in such a way as to get the prize. Everyone who competes in the games goes into strict training. They do it to get a crown that will not last; but we do it to get a crown that will last forever. Therefore I do not run like a man running aimlessly; I do not fight like a man beating the air. No, I beat my body and make it my slave so that after I have preached to others, I myself will not be disqualified for the prize.*
>
> –I Corinthians 9:24

Thank you, Lord, for focus, discipline, and consistency. Because even though it's a battle, the battle is not ours but the Lord's. All we need is a willing heart. With consistency, our bodies and minds will naturally elevate to new levels, and we will achieve the health and wellness goals set before us. I will not be disqualified for the prize in Jesus's name. And I pray.

Thank you, Lord, that I get the prize in Jesus's name. I beat my body and make it my slave. I control my body. I choose what to put in my mouth. I choose to work out. I choose the days that I work out and the time that I work out. I choose to be consistent.

I choose to walk in health and healing. If I fall off, I pick myself back up, and I keep pressing forward to the high calling in Jesus's name. The Lord chose to make my body in such a way that even if I break a limb, my body will quickly rush to heal. My body works to heal me every day. I drink plenty of water to stay hydrated, and the oxygen I breathe in heals me. He breathed the breath of life in me, and I became a living soul. I am alive! I see the results, I feel the results. I am walking/running toward my first goal of one year toward health and healing for the rest of my life. I get the prize. I can see the prize. I am close to the finish line, and I can feel the fever. Just the thought

Chapter Six: Devotion and Prayer

of making it to one year is motivating me and causing me to press on! I could not do this alone. I could only do this with the help of Jesus. I could only walk three to six miles with the help of Jesus. I could only run three to six miles with the help of Jesus. I could only walk or run a marathon and make it to the finish line with the help of Jesus. I keep going in the name of Jesus. I keep trying in the name of Jesus. My efforts are taking me to the finish line in the name of Jesus. I decree and I declare and command great health. I command healing. I command deliverance. I command a new hope. I command visions, I command dreams. I command strength. I command completion. Not abortion. I will not abort working out. I will not abort eating right. There is no aborting my dreams, visions, purpose. I walk in completion. I finish the race. I beat my body; the battle is not mine—it's the Lord's. I get the prize. I can see it, taste it, envision it in Jesus's name. I win! Amen.

Chapter Six: Devotion and Prayer

Thoughts for the month...

Journal your journey, the highs and the lows, it's all progress that will lead to your goals and your testimony. Journal what you eat, how you feel, your progress mentally, physically and spiritually and your thankfulness.

My Journal — Weeks 32-36

Weight: _____

Body Fat %:_____

Body Mass Index: _____

Measurements: Waist:_____ Chest:_____

    Hips:_____ Arms:_____ Legs:_____

What I eat: _____

_____

_____

_____

How I feel in body, mind and spirit:_____

_____

_____

_____

_____

What I am thankful for: _____

_____

_____

_____

Chapter Six: Devotion and Prayer

Prayer 10
Weeks 36-40

> *But blessed are the eyes because they see, and your ears because they hear. For I tell you the truth, many prophets and righteous men longed to see what you see but did not see it, and to hear what you hear but did not hear it.*
>
> –Matthew 13:13-17

Thank you, Lord, for the revelation to want to be healthy. To want to increase my worship and praise. I could have been lost in my sorrows and dead in my sins, but you opened the eyes to my heart so that I could see. And I pray.

I thank you, Lord, for vision. I thank you, Lord, that you have shown me the way to life. I thank you that you have allowed me the opportunity to feel your healing power in my body. I thank you, Lord, that when we ask you for something, you give us something to do. I thank you, Lord, that you have kept me healthy enough to make the change. I thank you, Lord, that you have made me a hearer and a doer of the Word. I thank you, Lord, that I heard you and you placed a burden on my heart enough to walk in the light. I thank you for the light. I feel great, Lord. I thank you, Lord. I thank you, Lord, that I am free. I thank you, Lord, that I am pressing forward and not looking to the right hand or to the left. I thank you that you are a lamp to my feet and a light to my path. I feel wonderful, Lord. I hear you, Lord. I can see you, Lord.

Your love is all over me, and everything that was incomplete in my life is coming into completion in Jesus's name. I'm stronger, I'm wiser, I'm better, I'm healthier, I'm whole, I am free of disease. I am free of depression. I am free of stress. I am free of confusion. My mind is clear. You put a smile on my face, Lord. I am free to worship, I am free to praise. I am free to love, I am free to encourage and be an example. I am no longer hidden in the closet; I am free. I am free to undergird, and I am free to lead. I am free,

Chapter Six: Devotion and Prayer

and I hear you, Lord. Let your will be done. Your way is my way. Thank you that I am encouraged. I see vision. I see growth. I am free. Amen.

Chapter Six: Devotion and Prayer

Thoughts for the month...

Journal your journey, the highs and the lows, it's all progress that will lead to your goals and your testimony. Journal what you eat, how you feel, your progress mentally, physically and spiritually and your thankfulness.

My Journal – Weeks 36-40

Weight: _____

Body Fat %: _____

Body Mass Index: _____

Measurements: Waist: _____   Chest: _____

   Hips: _____   Arms: _____   Legs: _____

What I eat: _____

_____

_____

_____

How I feel in body, mind and spirit: _____

_____

_____

_____

_____

_____

What I am thankful for: _____

_____

_____

_____

Chapter Six: Devotion and Prayer

Prayer 11
Weeks 40-44

> *Beloved, I wish above all things that thou mayest prosper and be in health, even as thy soul prospereth.*
>
> –III John 1:2

Prosperity and being in good health is the will of God. I meditate on that today. Increase is your will and your way, Lord! And I pray.

I thank you, Lord, that there is no such thing as good health or bad health, just health. Health and healing stand alone. I know that you wish the best for us, Lord, and right now I will let the motivation of my workout and nutrition fall into every area of my life. I work out and worship! Every area of my life is dedicated to you.

I walk and run in my purpose, I walk and run in my calling, I walk and run in my visions, I walk and run in my dreams, and all areas are done in the spirit of completion. Songs are being written, books are being completed, marriages are being restored, children are healthier and happier, ministries are being restored, churches are being healed. Hearts are purified, minds are clearer. Now I can practice patience. I will go on a mental fast. I will display a sweet spirit; I will be a blessing in the church. Bless me, Lord, to be a living example of the church. I want to walk right. I want to talk right. I want to be right. I want to live right. I give my body as a living sacrifice.

I thank you, Lord, that I am healed and that I am whole. I win, I walk in success. I win the prize in Jesus's name. I see the finish line. I thank you that this is the season to end and start again. I am at a higher level in Jesus's name. I will never stop eating healthfully; I will never stop working out. I thank you, Lord, that you have battled my disease. I thank you that I am achieving my goals. I thank you, Lord, for a new season. I feel great, Lord! Thank you. For you are the Lord, my healer! Amen!

Chapter Six: Devotion and Prayer

Lord my healer. I thank you Lord for a new season. For you are the Lord my healer. I feel great Lord, thank you…For you are the Lord my healer! Amen.

Chapter Six: Devotion and Prayer

Thoughts for the month…

Journal your journey, the highs and the lows, it's all progress that will lead to your goals and your testimony. Journal what you eat, how you feel, your progress mentally, physically and spiritually and your thankfulness.

My Journal – Weeks 40-44

Weight: _____

Body Fat %:_____

Body Mass Index: _____

Measurements: Waist:_____ Chest:_____

    Hips:_____ Arms:_____ Legs:_____

What I eat: _____

_____

_____

_____

How I feel in body, mind and spirit:_____

_____

_____

_____

_____

_____

What I am thankful for:_____

_____

_____

_____

Chapter Six: Devotion and Prayer

Prayer 12
Weeks 44-48

> *For though we walk in the flesh, we do not war after the flesh: (For the weapons of our warfare are not carnal, but mighty through God to the pulling down of strong holds;). Casting down imaginations, and every high thing that exalteth itself against the knowledge of God, and bringing into captivity every thought to the obedience of Christ.*
>
> –II Corinthians 10:3–5

Thank you, Lord, that I have reached my goal of working out for a full year! I can do all things through Christ, who strengthens me! And I thank you, Lord, that you have pulled down the strongholds, the imaginations, and any high thing that was holding me back from achieving all my healthy goals. Bless me, Lord, that, with my testimony, I can encourage everyone that I meet. And I love you, I praise you and thank you. And I pray.

I thank you, Lord, that I am completing a whole year of working out. I thank you, Lord, that you have pulled down the strongholds of laziness, tiredness, death, depression, confusion, bitterness, unforgivingness, bad eating, and all those things that had me bound. All those things that were blocking me from pressing forward to the high calling that you have provided for me. Thank you, Lord, that the weapons of our warfare are not carnal but mighty through the pulling down of strongholds. I thank you, Lord, that right now I cast down imaginations and every high thing that exalts itself against the word of God. I am the first and not the last, I am above and not beneath, I am a high priest a holy nation, a peculiar person in Christ Jesus. I can do all things through Christ, who strengthens me. I am a visionary, I am more than a conqueror; I am victorious, I am set free. I am strong in the Lord and in the power of his might. You said, "I am come that they might have life and that more abundantly" (John 10:10). I thank you because I AM is whomever we need you to be because you are El Elyon, above all circumstances and situations. You are Jehovah

Chapter Six: Devotion and Prayer

Rapha, my healer, and I thank you for my life and for Life—joy, peace, love, happiness, wholeness, kindness, gentleness, meekness, laughter, faith. I thank you, Lord, that I am truly pressing forward to a lifestyle of health and wholeness. I continue to work out, strengthen, and stretch. I continue to heal. I continue to ward off anything or any plague nigh my dwelling in Jesus's name. My knees are strong and stretched and lubricated, my hips are strong, my ankles are strong, my feet are strong, my back is strong, my shoulders are strong, my neck is strong, and my full skeletal and muscular frame is strong and stretched and lubricated.

I thank you, Lord, for a new level! I thank you, Lord, for completion! I thank you, Lord, that I have won the race and completed the course! I thank you, Lord, for victory! I am victorious and looking good and feeling good. And I will bless the Lord at all times, and his praises shall continuously be in my mouth! (Psalms 34:1). Amen.

Chapter Six: Devotion and Prayer

Thoughts for the month...

Journal your journey, the highs and the lows, it's all progress that will lead to your goals and your testimony. Journal what you eat, how you feel, your progress mentally, physically and spiritually and your thankfulness.

My Journal – Weeks 44-48

Weight:_____

Body Fat %:_____

Body Mass Index: _____

Measurements: Waist:_____ Chest:_____

   Hips:_____ Arms:_____ Legs:_____

What I eat: _____

_____

_____

_____

How I feel in body, mind and spirit:_____

_____

_____

_____

_____

_____

What I am thankful for:_____

_____

_____

_____

Chapter Six: Devotion and Prayer

A Prayer for You

If you do not have a relationship with God, this workout will still work for you. The principles of the Lord still stand, whether or not you know Jesus Christ as your Lord and savior. You may achieve physical health, but you may lack in spiritual health. This book exercises not only your body, but also your spirit.

The Bible says that *"if you believe with your heart and confess with your mouth that Jesus is Lord, you shall be saved"* (Romans 10:9). The Bible also says that *"if you ask anything in my name, I will do it"* (John 14:14). If you want to know the Lord, then you can simply pray this prayer and you shall be saved:

Dear Lord, thank you for dying on the cross for me. Thank you for forgiving me of all of my sins. Today I want to develop a relationship with you, Lord. I believe with my heart and confess with my mouth that you are Lord and savior of my life. I love you Lord … in Jesus's name I pray. Amen!

Now join a church and read the Bible to get to know the Lord better.

You are now saved! God bless you!

About the Author

For fourteen years, Lazet Michaels Boatmon has been a fitness professional. She is certified with the National Association of Sports Medicine (NASM) and Lazet is certified and experienced in:

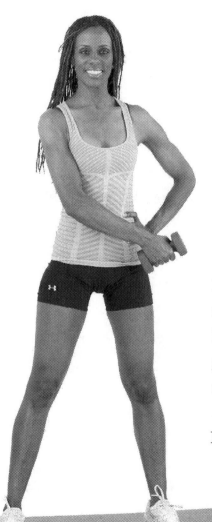

- Personal training
- Aerobics
- Step aerobics
- Pre/postnatal
- Boxing
- Cardio kickboxing
- Yoga sculpt
- Jazz dance
- Marathon training
- Teaching clients how to lose weight

Lazet is the owner of the Life Center private fitness facility in Detroit, CEO of the Persuaded Records gospel label, praise and worship leader, gospel artist, and executive producer and host of the exercise, health, and wellness television program *Working Out with Lazet*. Lazet is a resident of Detroit and New York.

Body Mass Index (BMI) Chart

	Underweight Below 18.5		Normal 18.5 - 24.9		Overweight 25.0 - 29.9		Obese 30.0 and above

BMI	Height (in)																		
Wgt. (lbs)	58 4'10"	59 4'11"	60 5'0"	61 5'1"	62 5'2"	63 5'3"	64 5'4"	65 5'5"	66 5'6"	67 5'7"	68 5'8"	69 5'9"	70 5'10"	71 5'11"	72 6'0"	73 6'1"	74 6'2"	75 6'3"	76 6'4'
100	21	20	20	19	18	18	17	17	16	16	15	15	14	14	14	13	13	13	12
105	22	21	21	20	19	19	18	18	17	16	16	16	15	15	14	14	14	13	13
110	23	22	22	21	20	20	19	18	18	17	17	16	16	15	15	15	14	14	13
115	24	23	23	22	21	20	20	19	19	18	18	17	17	16	16	15	15	14	14
120	25	24	23	23	22	21	21	20	19	19	18	18	17	17	16	16	15	15	15
125	26	25	24	24	23	22	22	21	20	20	19	18	18	17	17	17	16	16	15
130	27	26	25	25	24	23	22	22	21	20	20	19	19	18	18	17	17	16	16
135	28	27	26	26	25	24	23	23	22	21	21	20	19	19	18	18	17	17	16
140	29	28	27	27	26	25	24	23	23	22	21	21	20	20	19	19	18	18	17
145	30	29	28	27	27	26	25	24	23	23	22	21	21	20	20	19	19	18	18
150	31	30	29	28	27	27	26	25	24	24	23	22	22	21	20	20	19	19	18
155	32	31	30	29	28	28	27	26	25	24	24	23	22	22	21	20	20	19	19
160	34	32	31	30	29	28	28	27	26	25	24	24	23	22	22	21	21	20	20
165	35	33	32	31	30	29	28	28	27	26	25	24	24	23	22	22	21	21	20
170	36	34	33	32	31	30	29	28	27	27	26	25	24	24	23	22	22	21	21
175	37	35	34	33	32	31	30	29	28	27	27	26	25	24	24	23	23	22	21
180	38	36	35	34	33	32	31	30	29	28	27	27	26	25	24	24	23	23	22
185	39	37	36	35	34	33	32	31	30	29	28	27	27	26	25	24	24	23	23
190	40	38	37	36	35	34	33	32	31	30	29	28	27	27	26	25	24	24	23
195	41	39	38	37	36	35	34	33	32	31	30	29	28	27	27	26	25	24	24
200	42	40	39	38	37	36	34	33	32	31	30	30	29	28	27	26	26	25	24
205	43	41	40	39	38	36	35	34	33	32	31	30	29	29	28	27	26	26	25
210	44	43	41	40	38	37	36	35	34	33	32	31	30	29	29	28	27	26	26
215	45	44	42	41	39	38	37	36	35	34	33	32	31	30	29	28	28	27	26
220	46	45	43	42	40	39	38	37	36	35	34	33	32	31	30	29	28	28	27
225	47	46	44	43	41	40	39	38	36	35	34	33	32	31	31	30	29	28	27
230	48	47	45	44	42	41	40	38	37	36	35	34	33	32	31	30	30	29	28
235	49	48	46	44	43	42	40	39	38	37	36	35	34	33	32	31	30	29	29
240	50	49	47	45	44	43	41	40	39	38	37	36	35	34	33	32	31	30	29
245	51	50	48	46	45	43	42	41	40	38	37	36	35	34	33	32	32	31	30
250	52	51	49	47	46	44	43	42	40	39	38	37	36	35	34	33	32	31	30
255	53	52	50	48	47	45	44	43	41	40	39	38	37	36	35	34	33	32	31
260	54	53	51	49	48	46	45	43	42	41	40	38	37	36	35	34	33	33	32
265	56	54	52	50	49	47	46	44	43	42	40	39	38	37	36	35	34	33	32
270	57	55	53	51	49	48	46	45	44	42	41	40	39	38	37	36	35	34	33
275	58	56	54	52	50	49													

References:

Dr. Ian K. Smith M.D. 2006. *The Fat Smash Diet.* St. Martin's Griffin.

Cindy Trimm. 2007. *Commanding Your Morning.* Charisma House.

Don Colbert, M.D. 2009. *Eat This and Live!* Siloam.

National Academy of Sports Medicine (NASM)

American Council on Exercise (ACE)

American Heart Association

Cover design by: Rob Deane/Avima

Photography by: Rob Deane/Avima

Design and layout: Melinda Bylow

Make-up by: Dani Thompson divasplus@yahoo.com

Workout anytime with Lazet.

Get the DVD, *Working Out With Lazet* from the hit TV show.

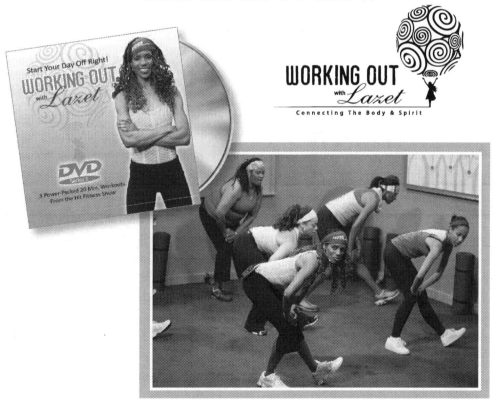

Get fit for life!

www.LAZETLIFE.com
866-94-LAZET